The or.   e
to making fat loss permanent

LOSE FAT FOREVER

Derek Alessi & Don Alessi Jr.

Clarence Bros. Press, Inc.
Williamsville, New York

Contents

Foreword   xiii

Introduction   1

Part I: The Truth

1   Never diet again!
       (Jamie the Dieter)   7
2   Let your lean muscle tissue burn your body fat
       (Karen the Toner)   15
3   Eat like a Viking!
       (Michael the Meal Skipper)   23
4   Burn, baby, burn!
       (Sandra the Calorie Counter)   29
5   Cheating is legal!
       (Chuck the Cheater)   37
6   All fat is not created equally!
       (Faye the Fat Eliminator)   41
7   Sugar warning!
       (Monica the Sugarholic)   47
8   Don't be fooled by slick marketers
       (Daryl the Duped)   61
9   Aerobic exercise can make you fatter
       (Mary the Aerobic Freak)   73
10   Spend less time in the gym
       (Mary the Aerobic Freak, Part Two)   79
11   Continuing the same workout will result in—nothing!
       (Jim the Burnout)   83
12   There is no such thing as the perfect time!
       (Dave—I'll start fresh next week)   89
13   Get help!
       (Rob the Type A Personality)   93

Part II: A New Life

14	Begin your transformation	103
15	Questions and answers	117
16	Words of encouragement	131

Part III: Time to Eat!

| 17 | Sample meal plans and grocery list | 141 |

Part IV: Body in Motion

18	Exercise instructions	151
19	The workouts	155
20	A visual guide to the exercises	187
21	Chart your progress	233
22	Maintain your success!	265

| Glossary | | 267 |
| Sources of information | | 273 |

DEDICATION

I would like to dedicate this book to all of the wonderful clients with whom I have had the privilege of working to shape their health and fitness over the years. Their trust in my system and me has helped us all to accomplish so much.

I would also like to dedicate this book to all of the well-intentioned individuals who want to improve their health and fitness, but have fallen victim to misleading information. You still have time to transform your life. In this book I will walk you through the transformation, step-by-step, that will improve your life permanently—as long as you stick with it and don't give up!

ACKNOWLEDGEMENTS

I believe that there is no greater job a person can have than to help enable a dedicated person improve his or her health and fitness. Throughout my career, I have had the great fortune of assisting people to dramatically transform their lives. This endeavor is both challenging and exciting, particularly for those of you who are about to read this book. I know that if you are committed to this program, you will be successful in achieving your goals.

Through the years, I have had help developing this program, as well as writing this book. I would like to acknowledge and thank the individuals who have aided me in this pursuit. They include first and foremost my family:

My brother and business partner, Don. We have battled body fat and helped teach and encourage individuals to take better care of their health and fitness for the past ten years. Don is constantly bettering himself through his tireless research of fitness principles. He was instrumental in developing the workout and exercise section of this system, as well as providing invaluable research. I consider Don the best personal trainer in the business.

My wonderful wife Andrea, who has been with me and supported me through all of the ups and downs; she is and will always be my biggest fan.

My mother and father have also been supportive of Don's and my pursuits in weight training and exercise, even years ago when they thought that we were going to kill ourselves with those weights in the basement!

I would like to thank my editors, Brenda P. Haughey, Ph.D. and Dorothy and Ray Miller. Thanks to them, this book is readable. Bonnie Shiesley and Robert Rivera, personal trainers at Alessi Fitness, also deserve thanks for their assistance with typing the book and gathering the research upon which it is based. Lastly, I would like to thank Robert "Bobby" Corey for his computer knowledge in allowing this book to seamlessly interact with our website.

DISCLAIMER

Lose Fat Forever is designed to provide information about increasing your health and fitness. It is solely for informational and educational purposes and is not intended to provide medical advice. You are advised to consult with your physician or health care professional prior to beginning any exercise or nutrition program or if you have any concerns about your health. Lose Fat Forever is intended for use by healthy individuals eighteen years of age or older. The author, Alessi Fitness Inc., and Clarence Bros. Press Inc. shall have neither liability nor responsibility to any person or entity with respect to any loss, damage or injury alleged to be caused directly or indirectly by the information contained in this system.

FOREWORD

The Commitment

I congratulate you on your decision to transform your current state of health and fitness. Whether your goal is to shape and tone your body, increase your strength or dramatically reduce your body fat, this system will help you be successful. I must first warn you: I will not tell you what you want to hear. Rather, I will tell you what you need to hear.

It doesn't matter if you are male or female. It doesn't matter if you are eighteen or eighty years old. It doesn't matter if you have ever been in shape before or ever stuck with an organized exercise plan for more than the two weeks after a New Year's resolution. You have the power to *transform* your health and fitness. You have the power to benefit from increased energy and productivity. You have the power to wear clothes that reveal your new shape. And you also have the power to increase your enjoyment of life.

First, let me tell you that I don't intend to waste your valuable time. The information I will be sharing with you is cutting edge technology. The system I propose will work *100 percent* of the time. However, you must first make a commitment to the system. I need you to commit your time and effort to this system exactly as it is presented. This system is just like your education in school (only more exciting!). The more you put into it, the more you'll get out of it. So, I encourage you *not* to begin this system unless you absolutely commit to:

- Dedicating yourself to improving your health and fitness
- Dedicating yourself to following and completing the system
- Dedicating yourself to becoming the best you have ever been

If you have the discipline and are committed, you will succeed.

The Promise

No one intentionally sets out to become fat, out of shape or unhealthy, just as no one sets out to become lonely, bald or broke. It "just happens." The reason it happens is because most people don't have a plan for maintaining and improving their physical selves. While many establish financial or career plans, they do not do so for their health and fitness because they don't perceive it as important.

Hundreds of people have told me they simply don't have the time to dedicate to their health and fitness. They claim they must focus all of their time and energy on their work. I promise if you do not make time for your health and fitness, you won't be able to work toward building your career or material wealth for long. You will either not have the strength and energy to cope with your highly stressful job and will suffer lack of production or, worse yet, you will become like hundreds and thousands of individuals who suffer each year from heart disease, stroke, diabetes (type two is ninety-five percent preventable) and hypertension.

I personally work with many wealthy clients who have neglected their health to build their wealth, and who then attempt to use their wealth to buy back their health. Often they are unsuccessful at reversing the effects of obesity, diabetes, heart disease, osteoporosis and chronic fatigue. Every one of these clients tell me the same thing: "I wish I would have taken better care of my health and fitness sooner." Ironically, they aren't able to enjoy the material wealth they sacrificed their health to attain.

My goal for this book is to educate you so that you know the truth about your health and fitness. I want you to know how your metabolism works and how to increase its effectiveness. I want you to know how certain foods react within your body. I want you to discover how an investment of just three hours—or 1.6 percent of the week—will dramatically improve your health and fitness.

I also want you to learn how to take control of your nutritional habits and not to be deceived by misleading food marketers. I want you to understand the fraud behind fitness claims and radical diets. I intend to teach you the basic tools you will need to empower yourself to take control of your body. Your self-confidence, self-respect and sense of personal control will increase if you adhere 100 percent to Lose Fat Forever.

No one ever said at the end of his or her life, "I wish I had spent more time at the office." Don't let the enjoyment of life pass you by. Take action on the information in this book and you will be well on your way to leading a healthier, happier and more productive life by following my system. Are you ready to begin?

Things do not change; we change.

—HENRY DAVID THOREAU

INTRODUCTION

Many of my clients over the past ten years have expressed skepticism about beginning a new fitness and weight loss system. These well-intentioned people have paid hard-earned money for weight loss solutions in the past and failed to gain any lasting results. This wasn't because they were unwilling to make the commitment. Rather, it was because the weight loss technology couldn't possibly deliver the benefits it promised.

Many dieters get stuck in what I refer to as the "fly trap." Think of a fly that is stuck inside your car. The fly thinks it can go right through the window, so it rams the window hoping to escape. Then, *wham!* It smashes itself against the window. After taking time to gather its wits, the fly crashes into the window once again, hoping to escape. And *wham!* The fly never learns. It keeps trying the same approach hoping for a different result.

The same thing happens when you go on a diet. You may have tried diets in the past on which you have lost weight initially, but then, *wham!* You still did not achieve the fitness or health results you wanted. Perhaps you even became fatter or more out of shape after the diet. So you tried another diet, hoping for a different outcome. As you have learned by now,

1

the end result of any diet will always be—*wham!* In Lose Fat Forever, I will show you why you cannot ever achieve lasting results through "dieting."

Perhaps you are similar to hundreds of clients with whom I have worked to transform their health and fitness. Before they begin their life-improving journey, they often ask me the following question: If this system works so well, why isn't everyone in great shape?

The answer is because it takes time and effort and, unfortunately, Americans are entangled in the quick-fix, instant gratification syndrome. They are misled into believing they can have whatever they desire in an instant, without making any sacrifices. Year after year, new *deceptive* products and programs hit the market promising to block fat, shape and tone your abs in three minutes a day, or promising that you can eat whatever fattening foods you want as long as you count the points. The common theme among these products is: it's quick, it's easy and it works like magic!

All of these strategies are intended to do one thing—convince you to believe in them and purchase their product. I don't want to sound negative, but you'll *never* reach the health and fitness level that you want by relying on these deceptive approaches. And it isn't because of you; it's because of them! These products and programs are not designed to produce results, and they will not work. They are designed to sell and make money! Do you think that infomercial companies are looking out for your best interest or theirs?

Pharmaceutical companies spend a fortune getting the Food and Drug Administration (FDA) to approve new "diet drugs" and "fat blockers" so that, as soon as the side effects are exposed to the general public, another product can instantly jump in as the next best seller. Food manufacturers have learned to manipulate labeling laws in order to capitalize on the American desire for better nutrition without delivering a better product. Nutritionists are getting their degrees from schools using textbooks that are sometimes more than twenty-five years old, the majority of which are written by food manufacturers. I've met more overweight and out-of-shape nutritionists and dieticians than in-shape and healthy ones.

Lose 30 pounds in 30 days! You see signs and advertisements like this everywhere. Now, would you be more likely to try a product that offers a thirty-day solution or one like Lose Fat Forever that offers a lifestyle solution? Most people want it *now*; they would buy the *thirty-second* solution if one were offered! However, they will always be disappointed and revert back to the same state of being frustrated with their bodies. Eventually, Americans must realize that instant gratification doesn't exist in the quest for better health and fitness, no matter what infomercials say. If a product claims that you can lose weight, develop your abs or live longer and the next words resemble "Quick," "Easy," "Works Like Magic," or "Instantly," you are about to hear a lie.

Each year, an estimated 300,000 deaths in the United States are attributed in part to obesity. This nation is the fattest it has ever been and an increasing percentage of the population is living a sedentary lifestyle. According to Claude Bouchard, author of *Physical Obesity and Activity*, "Sedentarism in overweight or obese persons increases the probability that they will be affected by the common morbidities of excess weight or that they will die prematurely."

Bouchard also elaborates on the consequences of common morbidities: "The current epidemic of obesity in children, adolescents, and young adults will translate later into unprecedented numbers of cases of type two diabetes, hypertension, cardiovascular disease, gallbladder disease, postmenopausal breast cancers, osteoarthritis at the knees, back pain, and physical and mental disabilities."

According to Foreyt and Goodrick's article, "The Ultimate Triumph Of Obesity," an estimated $100 billion is spent in the United States each year as a result of the direct and indirect costs of obesity. These authors predict that by the year 2230, *100 percent* of the adult population in the United States will be obese if the obesity rate continues to grow at the current pace!

It should also be noted that the physical fitness—or lack thereof—in parents greatly affects their children. In fact, R.C. Whitaker, in his paper, "Predicting obesity in young adulthood from childhood and parental obesity," states, "Parental obesity is reported to more than double the risk of adult obesity among both obese and non-obese children under ten years of age. And some of this influence is likely to be due to environmental as well as genetic factors." In other words, parents' health and fitness greatly affects their children's health and fitness.

If achieving good health and fitness were as easy as some advertisers lead us to believe, everyone should be in excellent shape. However, the Centers for Disease Control and Prevention published research documenting that sixty-one percent of Americans are overweight. This statistic is astounding given all of the health and fitness research that has been published, the number of health clubs and personal trainers that are available and the abundance of "healthy" foods on the market. This nation is in serious need of improvement. However, I'm not intending to help the entire nation with this book; I'm intending to help you. Follow this system daily and you will be in the best shape and fitness of your life!

PART I

THE TRUTH

■

1

NEVER DIET AGAIN!

Jamie, the dieter

Jamie came to me a few years ago wanting to shape and tone her body. She told me that her weight had gone up and down several times over the past two years. She said that she needed specific exercises to "spot" reduce areas of her body. I asked her what her primary goal was and she told me that she wanted to "lose weight." I asked her what kind of weight: muscle, water or fat? Jamie looked confused. No one had ever asked her this question before. She said, "Of course I want to lose fat. Who would want to lose just water weight?"

Next I asked her what activities she had tried to accomplish her goal. She said that she had joined a weight loss clinic a few years ago. I asked her about her experience with the clinic, and she said it was good. She lost seven pounds in the first ten days by cutting her calories to 1,500 per day.

She mentioned that she hit a minor plateau halfway through her second week of dieting. However, she met with her diet advisor (a non-degreed person paid by commission) at the clinic (a portly woman), who said it was "normal" to hit a plateau. The advisor then instructed Jamie to restrict her calories to 1,100 a day. She promised Jamie this would "jump start" her results. Jamie told me that she lost another five pounds but soon hit another plateau. Her advisor then told her she would have to lower her caloric intake to 950 calories a day to get to the next level!

Jamie said that, overall, the diet worked well. She lost more than seventeen pounds, but then she cheated. She craved the junk foods she had given up and she was tired of being hungry all the time. She wanted *more food*. Oddly enough, she was quick to point out that the diet had worked, but *she* failed!

I asked Jamie a simple question: "If initially you were losing weight at 1,500 calories a day, then had to cut down to 1,100 calories a day to lose weight, then eventually cut down to 950 calories, do you think that your metabolism was speeding up or slowing down?" I saw confusion on Jamie's face for a few seconds and then a look of shock. She said, "I must have slowed down my metabolism. Derek, I've heard that people can ruin their metabolism by dieting. Is it true?" I answered, "It is absolutely true."

When you diet by restricting calories, you condition your body to burn less fuel. The weight that you lose is water and lean muscle tissue. Remember, I asked Jamie what kind of weight she wanted to lose, muscle, water or fat. She answered "fat." However, "diets" are a short-term trick designed to lose water and lean muscle tissue. The long-term effect of "dieting" is a gain in body fat and a slower metabolism! And this was not the first time Jamie had dieted. In fact, she had lost and gained weight dozens of times before. Jamie was tired of living this "yo-yo" lifestyle.

My first recommendation to Jamie was to stop yo-yo dieting and hide her scale in the attic. Scale weight doesn't matter! If you develop good lean muscle tissue and are properly hydrated with water you will weigh more on the scale. Does this mean that you have gained fat? No! However, dieting gets rid of valuable lean muscle tissue and water while *retaining body fat!*

Never diet again!

Losing water weight can cause cell dehydration and muscle loss. When cell dehydration occurs, water should be replenished quickly by drinking additional water. However, you cannot afford to lose muscle tissue. The less muscle tissue you have, the less fuel

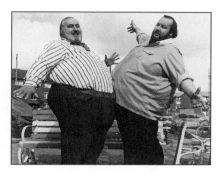

"Dieting" will ruin your metabolism!

(food) your body will burn. Since muscle is composed of roughly eighty percent water, the loss of water will lead to less muscle tissue. Hence, your metabolism will be slower and you will condition your body to become fatter.

Weight loss clinic regimens and various diets deceive you with an old trick: they get you to lose water quickly and thus your "scale weight" will be lower. However, you also lose good, valuable muscle and this is extremely detrimental to your fat-reducing goals.

The decrease in lean muscle tissue makes your body less efficient at processing food. At the end of the diet, you may very well be "lighter" on the scale, but your body fat percentage will likely be the same or higher than it was pre-diet.

In order to reveal this trick, I sometimes weigh my clients before a workout session. During and immediately post-workout, I make sure my clients consume at least twenty ounces of water. Upon re-weighing them, we learn that they have gained about two pounds. I then ask them, "Do you think you are two pounds fatter after the workout?" Of course not; it's just water fluctuation.

I recently conducted a corporate seminar for a Fortune 500 company educating their employees about how to take control of their health and fitness. The room was filled with more than 250 men and women. I began the seminar by asking the group, "How many people, by a show of hands, have ever been on a diet before?" Nearly every hand in the room went up. I then said, "How many people lost weight on the diet?" Once again nearly every hand went up. Next I said, "How many of you who lost weight, kept the weight off for good?" With nearly 250 people who claimed they lost weight on a diet, not one hand went up stating they kept the weight off for good. Lastly, I asked the group, "How many people here are in the best shape of their lives?" Once again, not one hand went up. I congratulated the group on their honesty, adding, "That's the same result as 99.9 percent of all people who ever diet. You never will keep the weight off for good because it is a mirage."

Think back to the last time you dieted. You may have lost "scale weight." In fact, you may even remember that your clothes fit better. However, did you feel that your metabolism was moving at a fast rate? Did you have the energy to work and play from dawn to dusk? Did you feel toned or flabby? Did you keep the weight off for good? Dieting is a yo-yo trap that cannot ever bring long term success. Restrict your calories and you will impair your metabolism and lose water weight.

Throughout my career, I've learned that most people don't like to diet. It isn't a pleasant experience to deprive yourself of food in exchange for the future hope of looking or feeling better. If you have ever dieted before, I'm sure you remember that you literally counted the days until it was over! Most people think of the pain of dieting the way they think of death. In fact, the first three letters in diet spell the word "die." Since dieting is an unpleasant and *ineffective* alternative, I am going to share with you a new technology that will work 100 percent of the time. I will show you the only no-nonsense guide to making fat loss permanent.

Let's start by defining an important term. When I ask most people to define metabolism, they usually start off by telling me how they can just look at a piece of cake and gain weight, while a friend or relative of theirs can eat whatever they want and never gain a pound. Metabolism is simply the rate or speed at which your body processes food. When your metabolism is fast, you will process food quickly. Unless you have a medical condition such as hypothyroidism, or are using certain medications, everyone can increase his or her metabolism.

I know this seems hard to believe, but you can absolutely take control of and choose the rate of your metabolism. You can condition your metabolism to process food at a staggering rate and you can burn more calories and eat more food than you ever dreamed possible. And you can do it without dangerous and expensive (soon to be banned) over-the-counter "metabolism increasing" drugs, without useless prescription "fat blockers" and best of all, without ever starving or going on a "diet."

The story about Jamie in the beginning of the chapter, like others I will share with you, is based on actual situations I have had with my clients over the years. However, their names have been changed to protect their privacy.

I don't blame Jamie—she was a victim of the diet industry. I want to believe that the weight loss clinic did not deceive her intentionally. They just didn't know any better and she was victimized by misinformation.

Commercials and infomercials are notorious for deception and misinformation. In fact, you may have seen a few of the various "miracle juice diets" on the market. They are available everywhere, including department stores, drug stores, grocery stores and even gas stations!

First, if a product claims it is a "miracle," you are about to hear a lie. Secondly, if a "diet" product professes a time frame such as "instantly," "overnight," "while you sleep," "48 hours" or "in 10 days," you are about to be deceived again. Next, if you take time to read the ingredients list, it is a mixture of juices, sugar and fruit extracts. That's it! I can guarantee that if you buy a "miracle juice diet," it will be the most expensive bottle of fruit juice you ever bought in your life!

Now, if you read the directions of any of these products, day one usually reads, "Mix half of your 'miracle juice diet' with an equal amount of cold water, and sip it throughout the day. Do not eat any food, but be sure to drink at least 8 glasses of water." For day two, the directions read, "Repeat." After day two, the directions read, "Now, weigh yourself. The pounds have disappeared like magic!" One label further states, "The Miracle Juice Diet will make you a winner." This is an absolute embarrassment.

I don't believe it is a miracle to lose "scale weight" when you do not eat for two days. In fact, remember the last time you were sick with the stomach flu and did not eat. You lost "scale weight" at a staggering rate. On the second day of being sick, you didn't jump off the toilet and exclaim, "It's a 48-hour miracle!" You realized the scale weight you lost was due to elimination and a loss of water and some muscle tissue. The intestines contain 12 to 20 pounds of matter. If you reduce the matter in your digestive track, your scale weight will be lower. However, you did nothing to lower your body fat or increase your metabolism permanently.

No one can ever lose body fat permanently by calorie restriction alone. The *only* way to increase metabolism and lose fat is by 1) developing lean muscle tissue through resistance training 2) increasing the frequency of eating supportive foods and 3) performing a moderate amount of cardiovascular exercise. I call this concept SYNERGY. I teach my personal fitness clients how to use SYNERGY to create the body of their dreams.

The word synergy, by definition, is the combined effect of two or more agents that is greater than the effect of the sum of the agents. For fitness purposes, I refer to synergy as the combined effect of the development of lean muscle tissue, the frequency of eating supportive meals and a moderate amount of cardiovascular exercise. When weight training and supportive nutrition are performed individually, they have a metabolic effect (increasing metabolism) of ten percent. When cardiovascular exercise is performed alone it has a metabolic effect of five percent. When these components are performed in unison, they have an enormous synergistic metabolic effect of thirty to forty percent! So the best metabolic effect and measurable results will occur when these components are performed together.

This book will teach you how to sensibly incorporate these three synergistic components into your life in order to *transform* your body and improve your health permanently.

Never diet again!

Synergy chart

Activity performed alone	Metabolic increase
Weight training	10%
Supportive nutrition	10%
Cardiovascular exercise	5%
Activities performed together	**30–40%**

SUMMARY

- If you want to reduce your body fat for the rest of your life, never diet again.

- Restricting calories or "dieting" will slow down your metabolism.

- When you "diet," you condition your body to burn less fat, fewer calories and lose water.

- SYNERGY means 1) developing lean muscle tissue 2) increasing the frequency of eating supportive meals and 3) performing a moderate amount of cardiovascular exercise.

2

LET YOUR LEAN MUSCLE TISSUE BURN YOUR BODY FAT

Karen, the toner

I am fortunate to own a private personal training center across the street from a large health club. One day, Karen came storming into my gym and asked to speak to me about training. I could see that she was agitated about something, but before I could speak she blurted out, "How many treadmills do you have here?" I playfully answered, "How many do you need?" She said that the reason she asked was because she was "sick and tired" of waiting for treadmills at the health club across the street. I asked her, "How often do you walk on the treadmill?" She answered, "Every day for about sixty minutes."

Karen was about thirty-five years old, five feet six inches, and I would estimate about 175 to 180 pounds. She was large for someone who worked out for an hour every day. I asked her to describe her fitness goals. She replied, "I want to shape and tone my body." I then asked her why she walked so much on the treadmill. She said, "I read somewhere that walking is the best exercise you can do for toning the body." I asked her if she had ever done resistance or weight training. She said,

"No, I'm big boned and I don't want to get bulky. I just want to *tone*."

I asked Karen how many years she had been doing all this walking. She said, "For about two years." Then I asked her, "How many years do you think it will take to lose the weight you want and tone your body by *just* walking?" She didn't have an answer. I said, "Unfortunately, Karen, it won't happen in 100 years!"

I spent the next hour explaining to Karen that the only way the body burns calories and fat is through lean muscle tissue. If you don't have much lean muscle tissue, you won't burn many calories. I also told her that lean muscle is not big and bulky, *it is lean!* In fact, muscle tissue takes up four times *less* space than fat tissue! I informed her that she didn't have to give up walking on the treadmill entirely, but she needed to incorporate weight training into her workout plan and *reduce* the time she spent walking.

Karen was skeptical at first. This new information was completely different than anything that she had ever heard or read in the tabloids at the checkout aisle before. She told me that everyone at the big health club across the street recommended walking more and doing weight training less. I asked her, "Were the people walking on the treadmill fatter or thinner than the people who were in the weight room?" Karen answered, "Now that I think about it, the people who were in the weight room were much thinner and had more muscle tone than the people who just walked." She added, "Yeah, but can this work for me?" I told her I PROMISE it will work.

That consultation took place more than four years ago. To this day, Karen still trains with me three times a week and her weight is a lean 145 pounds. More important than her scale weight, Karen reduced her body fat twelve percent and lost four dress sizes! She feels better and looks better than when she was in college. Finally, Karen no longer spends sixty minutes at a time on the treadmill. She incorporates weight training, supportive nutrition and a moderate amount of cardio-vascular training into a sensible lifestyle. Karen has finally *toned* her body.

Let your lean muscle tissue burn your body fat!

For you to dramatically take control of your health and fitness, it's important for me to share with you the reasons or science behind Karen's success. The only way to increase the amount of fat or calories your body can burn is by developing your lean muscle tissue through resistance training. I will constantly reiterate this concept throughout the entire book. If you only learn one thing from this book, it will be that your muscle tissue controls your metabolism and decreases your body fat. If you don't have much muscle tissue, you won't be able to burn enough fat.

Now let's define some common fitness terms. What is a calorie and what does it mean to burn calories? The definition of a calorie is the amount of heat that is necessary to raise one kilogram of water one degree Celsius. What the heck does that have to do with your metabolism? When you burn calories, you're increasing heat production within your body. The only place in the body that produces heat and, consequently, the only place that burns fat or calories is the muscles or, more specifically, the mitochondria of the muscle.

The mitochondria are the powerhouses or energy factories of the muscle. They are the components of the muscle that utilize energy and produce heat. If you increase lean muscle tissue, you will also increase mitochondria. Consequently, if you increase your lean muscle tissue, you increase heat production within your body. The process of heat production uses fuel and burns calories.

Resistance or weight training is the most effective way to develop lean muscle tissue. Bouchard, in *Physical Obesity and Activity*, states, "Interventions that increase the quantity of fat

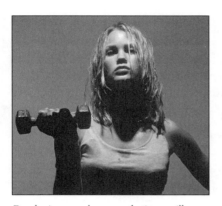

Developing your lean muscle tissue will increase your metabolism.

free mass [i.e., resistance training] may also increase fat oxidation and therefore be helpful in minimizing the increase in adiposity." In other words, when you increase your fat-free mass (muscle), you will increase the rate at which your body burns fat. Further, Bouchard states burning fat will decrease adiposity or body fat.

I consult with many clients like Karen, who initially believe they only need to perform cardiovascular exercise. Most of these individuals are women who want to shape and tone their bodies. When I first meet with them, I explain how their metabolism works. I teach them how muscle tissue uses energy and produces heat. Thus, much more fat is burned with weight training than with cardiovascular exercise. In fact, after a cardiovascular workout, your muscles will continue to produce heat and raise your metabolic rate for twenty minutes after you stop. Not bad! However, after a weight training workout, your muscles will produce heat and your metabolic rate will increase for up to seventeen hours! You can clearly see weight training is more efficient at burning fat and calories than cardiovascular training.

I encourage clients to try weight training and cut back on cardiovascular training. While most are apprehensive at first, after about four weeks they tell me that their clothes are fitting better. They usually ask, "But how can this be? I'm exercising less than before, but getting in better shape and reducing more body fat." The answer is simple: they allowed their bodies to gain lean muscle tissue.

As the body ages, muscles naturally atrophy, decreasing in size, strength and density. When muscle breaks down, there is less lean muscle tissue in the body. This is why I'm often asked, "How come I'm getting fatter each year? I'm not eating more or differently than in the past." The answer is because you have less muscle tissue than years earlier. In fact, after the age of twenty, for both men and women, the body naturally loses seven pounds of lean muscle tissue every ten years or .7 pounds of lean muscle a year. Once women reach menopause, muscle atrophy more than doubles! Their bodies lose upwards of fifteen pounds of muscle every ten years. This leads to loss of bone density and osteoporosis as well as increased body fat and a slower metabolism. Many women over forty-five years of age experience this phenomenon and have gained fat and lost muscle tone at a rapid pace. Is there any question that resistance training is needed?

Metabolism and muscle tissue are directly correlated. The more lean muscle tissue you have, the faster your metabolism will be. This doesn't mean that you have to look like a body-builder or Zena (the muscle chick) to speed up your metabolism. It simply means that you need more lean muscle tissue than you currently have.

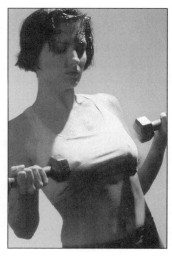

Muscle takes up four times *less* space than fat. For example, a pound of fat takes up about as much space as your clenched fist, whereas a pound of muscle takes up as much space as a silver dollar. So if you are worried that you will get bigger while exercising, you won't if you replace big bulky body fat with

Muscle takes up four times less space than fat!

lean tight and toned muscle. Lift weights and I promise you will not be disappointed with your results.

Developing lean muscle tissue is the single most important way to increase your metabolism. Muscle tissue in your body burns fat continuously, even when you are eating, watching TV, at work or sleeping. Increased muscle will speed up your resting metabolic rate (the rate at which you burn fuel while not exercising) and help you burn calories and fat twenty-four hours a day. In fact, for every pound of lean muscle tissue you add to your body, your metabolism will burn an extra fifty calories a day! So one added pound of muscle would burn 18,250 additional calories or five pounds of fat weight a year! If you were to add five pounds of lean muscle tissue to your body, you would burn an additional 91,250 calories or twenty-six pounds of fat a year!

For the purposes of this system, the primary benefit of developing lean muscle tissue is permanently increasing your metabolism and burning fat. Other benefits of weight training and developing lean muscle tissue include:

- Decreased LDL ("bad" cholesterol)
- Increased HDL ("good" cholesterol)
- Increased joint stability
- Improved bone density
- Improved balance
- Additional strength throughout the entire body
- Prevention of low back problems
- Improved glucose metabolism
- Improved posture and flexibility
- Reduction of high blood pressure
- Additional energy
- Better circulation
- Reduced stress

Let your lean muscle tissue burn your body fat!

20

SUMMARY

- When you develop lean muscle tissue, you produce heat, which has a metabolic effect of burning fat and calories.

- Increase your lean muscle tissue and you increase heat production within your body.

- The more lean muscle tissue you have, the faster your metabolism will work.

- Lean muscle tissue takes up four times less space than fatty tissue.

- Lift weights!

3

EAT LIKE A VIKING!

Michael, the meal skipper

When Michael called me for a consultation, his primary goal was to lose weight and increase energy. Michael was forty-six years old, five feet ten inches and weighed 220 pounds. Being a very successful attorney, Michael primarily worked behind a desk and performed little physical activity. Michael said he heard some wonderful things about me helping people drop fat, lose weight and regain their youth. I told him flattery would get him everywhere!

Michael told me that Jerry, a client of mine, referred him to me. He was impressed with how Jerry looked and how he was able to stick to his workouts with me for the past eighteen months. He said that Jerry had explained to him how important it was to do weight training and a moderate amount of cardiovascular training. Michael told me he understood how developing lean muscle tissue would increase his metabolism. He said he wanted to look and feel like a kid again, like Jerry. I said, "Great! It seems that Jerry is a good student and a great motivator." I asked Michael when he was able to begin his workouts and he said, "Tomorrow morning at 9 a.m." I asked him if he were planning on eating breakfast before the work-out and he said, "No, I never eat breakfast. I'm not hungry in the morning."

I asked Michael when he usually ate his first meal of the day and he said, "It depends. Sometimes I'm not hungry until dinner." I said, "If you want to speed up your metabolism, lose weight and feel like a kid again, it is important to eat fre-quently throughout the day." He asked me what "frequently" meant. I told him to eat every three to three and a half hours or five times a day.

Michael asked, "How am I going to do that? I'll gain weight and, besides, I'm not hungry during the day." I said, "You've gained weight just fine eating only once a day! If you eat the way I recommend, you'll lose fat rapidly." He said, "I understand the importance of eating frequently, but I'm just not hungry." I told him the reason he isn't hungry is because his metabolism is not burning fuel (food) efficiently. He isn't eating enough for the body to burn anything.

I also explained that his eating habits have conditioned his body to utilize less fuel, since infrequent meals will train the body to use as little fuel as possible. The body has an innate, fat-storing response to being starved. When the body feels starved, it slows down, burning fewer calories and expending less energy. This is why "dieting" doesn't work.

If you don't frequently nourish your body with supportive foods, your body will go into "starvation mode" and conserve energy and fat. You'll be unable to develop lean muscle tissue and increase your metabolism. Thus, you'll have little energy and a lot of body fat. Michael told me that no one had ever taken the time to explain it to him before. He just thought the less he ate, the less he would weigh. Unfortunately, this is how many individuals are *deceived* by the weight loss industry.

Michael began eating frequently. He has been one of my very best clients for the past three years and has transformed his waist from a hefty size forty to a slim thirty-four. He lowered his scale weight from 220 pounds of fat and jiggle to 185 pounds of ripple. He also increases his self-esteem to the point where he said, "I can now comfortably take my shirt off when I'm doing yard work!"

Eat like a Viking!

I tell many of my clients to "eat like a Viking." I don't mean you have to eat without utensils and stuff globs of fatty meats, cheeses and a drumstick into your mouth with dirty hands while Nordic warriors are fighting to the death. Rather, make sure you are eating supportive foods frequently. You'll be surprised how much food you can actually eat with this system while drastically reducing your body fat. You'll no longer have to resort to eating like a rabbit, consuming only celery, lettuce and carrots. Also, you will *never* have to starve yourself again.

Remember, metabolism is the speed at which your body uses fuel and processes food. Dieting or not eating will cripple your metabolism. If you want your body to get well-conditioned to burning food, it's very important to put food into the fat burning machine frequently. Also, the lean muscle tissue you are diligently working to increase needs small frequent meals to develop.

I know many people are initially afraid of eating frequently. This is because they have dieted before and think the diets have worked, but they have failed. Many of my clients are convinced if they increase meal frequency, they will gain weight. Well, guess what? Initially, they will! However, once they understand why, they will see this as something very positive.

In the last chapter, you learned why muscle is the single most important factor in increasing metabolism and burning fat. However, your bathroom scale cannot differentiate between good muscle weight and water, bone, fat, and internal organs. The scale just lumps them all together and gives you a grand total. In fact, if you were to cut off your arm

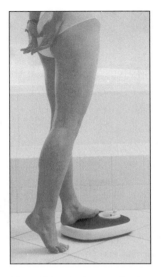

You will lose inches, not "scale weight," during the first month.

(please don't) you would weigh less on the scale. It sounds silly, but some people would actually be thrilled to see their scale weight go down! Using the scale is an awful indicator of your actual body composition and progress. Please, hide, break or give away your scale. It will do more harm than good.

When you develop muscle tissue, your scale weight will increase. Does this mean you are fatter? Absolutely not! You'll be leaner! You've heard before that muscle weighs more than fat. In fact, muscle tissue is 2.2 times more dense than fat. In other words, it is more than twice as heavy! I usually tell my clients not to expect to lose any scale weight during the first month of my system. However, you *will* lose fat and inches around your body.

Now, relax. Even though I don't want you to become preoccupied with it and even though it is a poor indicator of your progress, you will eventually lose scale weight. In fact, you may very well lose a lot of scale weight, depending on the condition you are in when you start this program. However, I want you to focus on body fat reduction and clothing sizes; they will lead you in the right direction. Your scale weight will follow your body fat and your clothing size. If you focus on your scale weight, your metabolism will most likely be slower and your body fat will remain higher. Trust me, I've seen these simple techniques work for hundreds of people over the past ten years.

Remember, if you lose weight and that weight is primarily water and muscle, your new lower weight will be short-term and unhealthy. Your objective is to maintain and increase your lean muscle tissue and water while ridding your body of fat.

Weight training is the only way to build lean muscle tissue and increase metabolism.

Now, to get back to meal frequency, the food or fuel you put into your body will be either supportive or not supportive of what you are trying to accomplish in the gym. If the body needs more fuel because of the additional muscle, you need to nourish the body with additional supportive fuel. This will increase the metabolic (fat-burning) effect of the muscle and overall metabolism will increase.

With my clients, I use an analogy comparing their metabolism to a fireplace. A fireplace burns fuel and produces heat just like our bodies do. It's easy to understand that if you don't put any logs on the fire, you won't produce any heat. The same is true for the body. If you eat infrequently, your body will not have any calories to burn. Conversely, if you put too many logs on the fire at the same time, you'll douse the flame and it will take a long time to burn through the wood. If you tend to binge eat and consume a lot at one time, you'll douse your metabolism and it will take a long time to burn through food.

Now, follow me and I will get you out of the fire for good! If you frequently put a few logs on the fire and let them burn, you will produce a flame with much heat. If you eat every three to three and a half hours, your body will produce additional heat and the frequent nourishment will support the development of your lean muscle tissue. When you do this in combination with resistance training (which acts like a bigger fireplace) and a moderate amount of cardiovascular exercise (which acts like quick lighter fluid), fat will be incinerated from your body!

The types of food you consume are also very important. I suggest you eat a supportive meal frequently. (By the way, I have scientifically concluded that it's more pleasurable to eat whole foods than to starve on low calorie, tinfoil wrapped diets!) I define a supportive meal as a serving of foods that contain a lean protein source, a slow-releasing carbohydrate (described later in the text) and a vegetable (preferably green).

It's that simple! If you eat three meals a day in this supportive manner and eat a snack between breakfast and lunch and between lunch and dinner, you will decrease your body fat rapidly. A snack or meal between your major meals should be smaller in size and calories (more about that later).

I know what you're thinking: you think I'm as crazy as all of the characters on late night infomercials! How can you possibly eat vegetables with every meal? Let me clear up this question and regain your trust. I don't expect you to eat green vegetables every morning, although some are great in omelets. I do expect you to eat vegetables at least twice daily. I recommend you eat vegetables with your lunch and always with dinner. I'll elaborate on various types of supportive foods later in the book.

Eat like a Viking!

SUMMARY

- Eat a supportive meal every three to three and a half hours.

- The more frequently you eat, the more conditioned and efficient your body will become at burning food.

- A supportive meal contains a lean protein, a slow-releasing carbohydrate, and a vegetable (preferably green).

4

BURN, BABY, BURN!
THE THERMAL EFFECT OF FOOD

Sandra, the calorie counter

Sandra was a doctor who had been working with me for about three months. She had made some wonderful gains lowering her body fat, increasing lean muscle tissue and energy. However, she wanted to bring her body to the next level. She wanted to dramatically lower her body fat and, to use her words, "rip up!"

I congratulated Sandra on her commitment. It's a nice feeling for me to watch people become passionate about their health and fitness. Only three months ago, Sandra had been hesitant about spending any time working out. In fact, when we first met she told me, "You know, I'm a doctor. It's difficult for me to commit to a dedicated program because I get paged for emergencies all the time." I replied, "Sandra, I know that you're busy, and I know that often you don't have control over your schedule. However, I can guarantee if your body is important to you, you'll never regret working with me to improve it." Sandra said, "Okay, I'll give it a try." Now, three months later, she wants to "rip up." I must be a better motivator than I thought!

Sandra asked me, "What will I have to do to rip up?" I replied, "You'll have to continue to weight train three times a week, perform cardiovascular training twenty to thirty minutes five times a week and eat supportive meals every three to three and a half hours." She said, "No problem. But how many calories should I eat?" I said, "Don't count calories. Just make sure that each serving is the size of your clenched fist." For example, a supportive meal is a fist-sized lean protein source, a fist-sized slow-releasing carbohydrate and a fist-sized green vegetable.

Sandra asked, "Why should I do that? Calories are calories." I explained to her that a lean protein source is essential to help repair and develop lean muscle tissue, a slow-releasing carbohydrate helps ensure the body has a stable energy supply, and green vegetables are a great source of insoluble fiber, which aids in digestion and general health. Sandra said, "Fine, that's all good, but to rip up, *calories* are still all the same."

I told Sandra that different macronutrients, proteins, carbohydrates and fats have different thermal effects, which means each macronutrient needs a different amount of energy for digestion. For example, protein contains the most complex molecular structure, composed of amino acids in clusters of twenty-two. The body must break apart amino acids into di- and tripeptides. Consequently, this requires a lot of energy or calories to digest. Fats, on the other hand, are extremely easy for the body to digest and don't use much energy or calories in digestion. Carbohydrates use more energy than fats, but less than protein.

Sandra was shocked to hear this. She never learned this in medical school. I wanted her to understand clearly that her body burns calories while it digests food. It burns the most calories eating lean protein sources and the least amount eating fatty foods. I wasn't suggesting she only eat protein, however, I wanted her to recognize that protein has the highest thermal effect of any food group.

Maybe you didn't know the reason why, but you instinctively knew that eating 1,000 calories of ice cream or 1,000 calories of lean chicken, brown rice and green beans isn't the same. Even though they are both 1,000 calories, your body will process and utilize them differently. This is another reason why dieting doesn't work. Even if you stay within your caloric intake (or points) on the diet, your body will utilize foods differently.

Sandra, still somewhat apprehensive, began to follow my advice. She wasn't disappointed. Within three months, Sandra slashed her body fat from nineteen percent to twelve and a half percent. She dropped three dress sizes and could finally see toned muscles. Her abdominals were defined. Sandra was ripped!

Your fitness goal may be the same as Sandra's, or you may only want to reduce your body fat minimally. While portion size is important, *do not* count calories. It is more important to your results to realize how your body utilizes food sources. Once you understand this concept, you will be on your way to achieving your fitness goals.

Burn, baby, burn!

Perhaps no one has ever taken the time to explain to you that food has a thermal effect. This means that it requires calories or energy to be processed and burned. Some foods require more calories or energy than others to break down and digest. The foods that require the greatest amount of energy to be utilized by the body are proteins. Protein has a thermal effect of twenty to twenty-five percent, which means if you consume 100 calories of protein, the thermal effect will burn twenty to twenty-five calories. The net effect in your body will only be seventy-five to eighty calories.

The thermal effect of carbohydrates is in the middle. All carbohydrates are not the enemy. While carbohydrates have gained a negative connotation recently thanks to some radical diets on the market, you still need to consume some because they are vital to your health and energy. Complex carbohydrates have a double peptide bond and typically take longer to break down and be released into the body. Examples of complex carbohydrates are pasta, potatoes, and rice.

Alternately, simple carbohydrates have a single peptide bond (you won't be tested on this) so they are broken down and released into the body more rapidly. Examples of simple carbohydrates are table sugar, candy, fruit and honey. In terms of lowering your body fat, these *are* the enemy. I usually recommend eating simple carbohydrates only on "cheat days." I will elaborate more on this later.

Complex carbohydrates have a thermal effect of ten percent. So if you consume 100 calories of what I term a "slow-releasing carbohydrate," such as brown rice, oatmeal or a sweet potato, you'll burn ten calories in the breakdown of these foods. The net result is ninety calories. I'll discuss the difference between slow- and fast-releasing complex carbohydrates in Chapter 7.

Fat has the lowest thermal effect at five percent. If you consume 100 calories of fat, five calories will be burned in the process. That leaves ninety-five calories remaining to either be utilized as energy or stored as body fat. Thus, it is easy to see that there is more to consider than just counting calories or grams of any particular food.

Thermal effect of food

Food	Thermal effect
Protein	20–25%
Complex carbohydrates	10%
Fats	5%

The following table lists most supportive foods. Included are lean protein sources, slow-releasing carbohydrates and vegetables.

Supportive Foods

Lean proteins	Slow-releasing carbohydrates	Vegetables
Egg whites	Wheat bread	Broccoli
Egg Beaters	Wheat pasta	Spinach
Chicken breast	Sweet potatoes/yams	Green beans
Turkey breast	Oatmeal	Asparagus
Steak	Brown rice	Mushrooms
Fish	Wild rice	Cauliflower
Shellfish	Whole grain couscous	Leafy lettuce
Cottage cheese (1%)		Peppers
Ostrich		
Pork		
Veal		
Buffalo (not the city)		
Tuna		
Protein powders		
Tofu		

Another question clients usually ask is, "How much should I eat at one time?" I doubt that you really want to get into the process of weighing or measuring all of your foods before you eat. The simplest way to ensure you are consuming the appropriate serving size of food is this: each portion should be the size of your clenched fist. For example, a supportive meal would be a fist-sized chicken breast, a fist-sized portion of broccoli and a fist-sized amount of brown rice. If you use your fist as a guide, you will always know how much to eat. Snacks eaten between major meals should be smaller in size and contain fewer calories. Reduce the serving size to approximately one-half clenched fist to satisfy this requirement or, for convenience, a good protein shake (more on this later).

I occasionally work with clients who are vegetarians. The challenge with these clients is to ensure they eat enough lean protein sources. Every one of these individuals I have worked with had a small amount of muscle tissue and high body fat. They usually lack vital amino acids, the building blocks of pro-

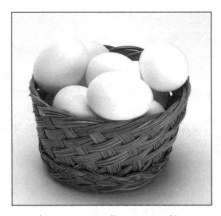

Egg whites are an excellent source of lean protein.

tein, and the development of muscle tissue is difficult at best without adequate protein for the recuperation and repair of muscle tissue.

If you are a vegetarian for religious or ethical reasons I'm not asking you to alter your commitment. However, if you are a vegetarian because you believe it is a "healthier" way to eat, I encourage you to re-examine your eating practices. I don't believe having a lack of protein and essential amino acids, high body fat and a low amount of lean muscle tissue is necessarily healthier. According to Joyce Forte in her article, "Vegetarians Versus Meat Eaters," "Vegetarians overall run a high risk of incomplete nutrition, but vegans (no meat, eggs, dairy, gelatin or honey) run the highest risk of incomplete nutrition as important vitamins and minerals are omitted from their diets."

If you are a vegetarian and willing to drink protein shakes (see Chapter 14), it's possible for you to consume an adequate amount of protein. This will help with the development of lean muscle tissue and the reduction of body fat without eating animal products. If you are unwilling to consume protein shakes, your development of muscle tissue will be difficult at best and your body fat will remain high. Remember, protein contains vital amino acids, vitamins and minerals your body needs to function properly.

Burn, baby, burn!

SUMMARY

- Fats are high in calories and have little thermal effect.

- Compared to fats, complex carbohydrates are lower in calories, provide useful energy and have a greater thermal effect.

- Proteins are essential and provide twice as much thermal effect as carbohydrates or fats.

- Protein is necessary for the development of lean muscle tissue and ridding the body of fat.

- You don't have to be perfect. I know that there will be times that you don't eat five small meals each day. I just ask that you follow this system as closely as possible. As I mentioned in the beginning of this book, the more effort you put into this system, the more you will get out of it.

5

CHEATING IS LEGAL!

Chuck, the cheater

Chuck was in his early fifties, and a large man. He had tried many different ways to lose weight and feel better including weight loss centers, fad diets and health clubs, but none of these methods worked for him. Chuck felt hopeless. He told me, "I need a solution that will work for good. No more quick fixes!"

Chuck was following my system well and didn't have any problem eating frequently or eating foods in the correct proportions. I was proud of him. I also discovered that he was an animal in the gym! He wasn't as strong as he had been in his twenties and thirties, but he worked out with more intensity than the next two people combined. He really wanted to improve his health and fitness.

Chuck was initially hesitant when I told him to use a "cheat day." He felt he should eat well all the time, and believed a cheat day would sabotage his results. I told him how important it was both mentally and physically to spend one day a week, eating whatever he desired in moderation. It's a great way to "reset" your system.

Chuck started using the cheat day and began to enjoy the concept. He would eat well all week long and then reward himself on Sunday with wherever he desired. He told me, "This isn't a bad system after all!"

Chuck began to see and feel results. He lost inches around his waist, his clothes fit better and he was able to move with less pain in his joints and muscles. He was thrilled!

However, Chuck began to stray from the system a few months later. He no longer used a cheat day. Instead, he spread out his cheat day over many days. He rationalized if he had a "cheat" lunch on Tuesday, a "cheat" dinner on Thursday and some "cheat" drinks during happy hour on Friday, it would be the same as combining them all on one day.

I became aware of this behavior during our monthly testing session. I regularly perform tests that include taking a percentage of body fat, girth measurements and lean body mass. Chuck's results had consistently been positive for two straight months. However, his results were negative this month. His body fat percentage and girth measurements had increased.

Chuck had still been attacking his workouts with intensity, so I knew that he didn't need a kick in the butt to increase his motivation. Upon examining Chuck's nutrition in detail, I recognized the cheating problem. He explained his rationale. He was having three to four cheat days a week and his body was suffering the consequences. It was time to explain to Chuck why this behavior was detrimental.

I told Chuck that his current eating behavior was "trapping" fat on his body. He was still working out hard, but his nutrition was not supporting the development of his lean muscle tissue. The frequency of his cheating was prohibiting his body from consistently utilizing his fat for energy. He was consuming too much simple sugar and spiking his insulin too frequently to lose fat.

Chuck appreciated this new information. In fact, he made me a promise. He said, "Now that I know what I did wrong, I will consistently drop fat every month."

Since the time Chuck modified his cheat days and made his promise, he dropped his waistline a massive five inches in just four months! Also, he lowered his body fat by 5.5 percent and increased his lean body mass by eleven pounds. His jacket went from size fifty-four to forty-six. Chuck was ecstatic. He learned how to use his cheat day properly and reaped the rewards.

Cheating is legal!

Clients have often asked me, "Can I ever eat the desserts and rich foods I love?" Absolutely! I believe that it is very important to eat whatever you enjoy or crave. If you deprive yourself of any type of food altogether, you will binge sooner or later and compromise your efforts. I recommend that you take one day a week and make it your cheat day. Just *one* day!

On your cheat day, eat whatever you desire, in moderation. For example, eat a piece or two of pizza, but not the whole pie. Eat a piece of cake, but not the whole sheet. It is still *very important* to eat frequently on your cheat day. You don't want to slow down your metabolism.

I've had some clients who initially say, "I don't need a cheat day; I'll be perfect all the time." I strongly warn you against not taking your cheat day. Sooner or later (we're all human) you will break down and binge.

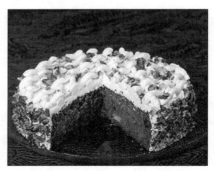

It's important to eat whatever you like, in moderation, one day a week.

I've seen clients go more than two months of eating perfectly, and then all hell breaks loose. They have deprived themselves so much they can rationalize eating anything. They get off their "game plan" and sometimes never recover.

Please use your cheat day to let off some steam and pressure. When you eat poorly after you have consistently eaten supportively, you'll feel awful and look forward to the next day when you can eat supportively again. I encourage you, use your cheat day.

If you want to continue to burn fat quickly and efficiently, limit your cheat day to one specific day each week. For example, make every Saturday or Sunday your cheat day. I recommend that you use one day on the weekend as a cheat day because it is usually easier to eat more supportively during the week when you are on a schedule.

Cheating is legal!

SUMMARY

- Incorporate one "cheat day" into your supportive eating habits.

- On your cheat day, eat whatever you want, in moderation.

- Meal frequency is still important even on your cheat day.

6

ALL FAT IS NOT CREATED EQUALLY!

Faye, the fat eliminator

Faye was one of the most genuinely nice clients I've ever had the privilege of working with. She worked hard at everything she did in the gym because athletics didn't come naturally to her. Faye, like many clients, was primarily interested in losing body fat and shaping her body.

When I work with new clients I typically begin their first two to three weeks by focusing on weight training, a moderate amount of cardiovascular training and eating small frequent meals. This initiates their development of lean muscle tissue and speeds their metabolism. Faye worked very hard and was progressing nicely in this introductory phase.

The next phase of my system introduces more detailed nutritional education. Faye understood the importance of eating small frequent meals. She knew this would speed up her metabolism. She also knew the significance of combining a lean protein source, a slow-releasing carbohydrate and a green vegetable into each meal. The only question that Faye had was, "How many grams of fat should I eat a day?"

I answered Faye by asking a question: "What kind of fats are you referring to—saturated, unsaturated or essential fatty acids?" She didn't know the difference between them and, like many, had read in the news that fat is bad. In fact, it has been promoted, mostly by food manufacturers, that fat must be eliminated altogether in order to lose weight and live "healthier." Unfortunately, nothing could be further from the truth.

I explained to Faye that all fat is not the same. Obviously, the fat found in doughnuts isn't the same and isn't as beneficial to you as fat found in freshwater fish like salmon or swordfish. *All* fat is high in calories and contains nine calories per gram. Remember, protein and carbohydrates contain just four calories per gram. However, the body uses saturated and unsaturated fat differently. The body doesn't have much use for saturated fat. It's the "bad" fat that clogs arteries. On the other hand, the body does have a need for unsaturated and, more specifically, polyunsaturated essential fat. These omega fats include flax oil, fish oil and safflower oil. This is "good" fat that

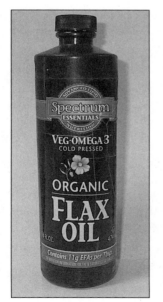

Flax oil is a great source of essential fatty acids.

is necessary to help you achieve your health and fitness goals.

The reason these fats are called essential fatty acids is because the body doesn't make them naturally. If the body doesn't get these fats from foods, lean muscle tissue will be broken down to get them. As you know, lean muscle tissue is important. If lean muscle tissue is broken down, your metabolism will work slower. This would be detrimental to your results, as it was to Faye's.

I recommended that Faye avoid saturated fat and hydrogenated oils (solid at room temperature) such as butter, peanut butter, margarine and vegetable oil. I also suggested she take a serving of flax oil daily.

These essential fatty acids help protect lean muscle tissue, control sugar cravings and regulate insulin.

Faye discovered how various fats react differently within the body. She also learned the importance of essential fatty acids and how they help protect lean muscle

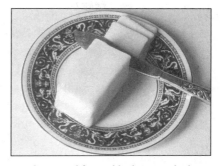

Avoid saturated fats and hydrogenated oils.

tissue. After she incorporated good fat into her nutritional program, she proceeded to drop her body fat by thirteen percent in ten months. She also gained more muscle tone and increased her energy level to the point where she felt like a kid again!

All fat is not created equally!

Americans have heard for the past fifteen years that they should limit fat intake, especially saturated fats. Notice that I said *limit* intake, not eliminate fat altogether. This is because fat is an *essential* macronutrient. The word essential means that dietary fat is necessary for basic processes of the body to occur and the body cannot produce these fats by itself.

I strongly recommend that my clients consume flax or fish oil daily. These essential fatty acids (EFAs) contain omega oils, specifically omega-3, which help stabilize blood sugar and provide a satisfied or satiated feeling to the mind and body. This will facilitate the reduction of sugar cravings and help complete the amino acid (protein building block) chains necessary for the regeneration of lean muscle tissue.

It is important to limit *saturated* fats like butter and lard, as well as fatty cuts of meat. It is also important to stay away from "hydrogenated" oils such as those contained in most peanut butters and margarines. These foods don't contain essential fatty acids. The body can easily make saturated fats from carbohydrates. Therefore, it isn't necessary to consume saturated fats. You should avoid them whenever possible, for they aren't supportive of a lean, toned and healthy body.

Remember, even though some fats are essential, fats are still high in calories. For example, one gram of fat equals nine calories, while one gram of carbohydrates and protein has just four calories. Also, as discussed earlier, fats have a low thermal effect. The calories of fat that you consume are not utilized as efficiently as proteins and complex carbohydrates in the breakdown of food.

Incorporating EFAs (good fats) into your nutrition will benefit both your health and fitness. You will feel better and lower your body fat.

Calories per gram of specific macronutrients

Proteins	4
Carbohydrates	4
Fats	9

All fat is not created equally!

SUMMARY

- All fats are not the enemy.

- The body requires essential fatty acids (EFAs) such as flax and fish oils, *not* saturated fats and hydrogenated oils.

- One gram of fat contains nine calories.

- One gram of protein or carbohydrates contains just four calories.

7

SUGAR WARNING!

Monica, the sugarholic

Monica was in her late fifties and new to exercise. Her primary goal was to lose "a lot" of weight, as she was about five feet nine inches and 260 pounds. She told me that she had been active most of her life enjoying golf, tennis and skiing, but when she hit forty-five years old, her metabolism and her activity level, just seemed to stop. She told me nutrition was not a problem because she ate "right." She then said she would follow any type of exercise training I recommend.

I've learned to question everything. If someone tells me they have been active and exercising I want to know what kind of exercise and how often. If someone says they eat "right," I want to know how they define eating right. I asked Monica to describe to me her typical day of nutrition.

She started off by telling me she eats a raisin and bran cereal with a banana and orange juice for breakfast every morning. She sometimes has an apple for a snack between breakfast and lunch. For lunch she usually has a sandwich with low fat turkey or ham and fat free cheese on a roll. For dinner she eats pasta or chicken and rice or some type of meat and potato. I asked her if she snacks after dinner and she said, "Sometimes, but always low fat products like cookies or pretzels."

Before I criticize or comment on someone's nutrition, I always ask, "How important is it for you to lose fat and regain your health?" Monica said, "It's very important." I asked, "Are you willing to do what it takes to accomplish your goals?" She replied, "Yes, whatever it takes." I said, "The primary reason you have gained so much body fat and weight over the last few years is for two reasons. First, as the body ages it loses muscle tissue and, consequently, your metabolism slows down. Secondly, you are eating about eighty to ninety percent of your calories from sugar!"

Monica thought and then said, "I never eat candy or drink soda pop. How can I be eating too much sugar?" I proceeded to describe the three primary macronutrients: protein, carbohydrates and fats. I emphasized to Monica that *all* carbohydrates are sugar. However, the body uses simple carbohydrates and complex carbohydrates differently. Simple carbohydrates like juice, candy, fruit and soda pop immediately spike blood sugar levels and cause an insulin response. Also, most enriched carbohydrates like white rice, white pasta and white bread also spike blood sugar levels because they are enriched with sugar.

I explained to Monica that the cereal, fruit, bread, pasta, juice, pretzels and low fat cookies are all *loaded* with enriched sugar. I didn't tell her to eliminate these foods forever. I just wanted her to understand that these foods won't help to lower body fat, lose scale weight or even increase long-term energy.

Complex carbohydrates and, more specifically, slow-releasing complex carbohydrates that contain no enriched sugar don't spike blood sugar levels as much or quickly. Therefore, slow-releasing complex carbohydrates don't cause as much of an insulin response. This helps the body sustain long-term energy and utilize fat more efficiently.

I recommended to Monica that she begin to replace simple carbohydrates and enriched white carbohydrates with slow-releasing carbohydrates like wheat pasta, brown rice and wheat bread. Next, I recommended the reduction of all carbohydrates, including slow-releasing ones, to approximately forty percent of her caloric intake. This percentage may vary per individual dependant upon goals, physical condition and age.

Lean protein sources and green vegetables should replace the excess amount of carbohydrates in her daily eating habits. I reiterated the importance of eating a lean protein source, a slow-releasing carbohydrate and a green vegetable every three to three and a half hours.

Finally, I insisted that Monica must continue to weight train and perform a moderate amount of cardiovascular training three times a week. Remember, lean muscle tissue is the only place in the body where fat and calories are burned. Since Monica is post-menopausal and has lost considerable lean muscle tissue, weight training is essential for the achievement of her goals.

Monica is continuing to work hard to meet her goals, and is still a work in progress. She currently has reduced her body fat five percent in four months and has lost twenty pounds of scale weight. She knows she has a long way to go and is committed to attaining results. I continuously encourage Monica to work hard, eat well and be patient. She's doing better every day.

Sugar warning!

Simple carbohydrates (sugar) are a different concern from fat altogether. The consumption of sugar is necessary for energy. However, I've seen hundreds of clients dramatically transform their bodies by avoiding most simple and some complex sugar. I've read agricultural reports that indicate the average

49

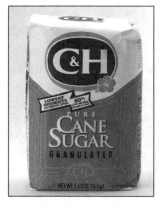
Limit your sugar consumption.

American consumes between 150 to 180 pounds of sugar per year! And that's what the *average* American consumes. Just think how much sugar those who are not aware or careful of their nutrition consume in a year!

Whenever you consume sugar, whether simple or complex, your blood sugar level will increase. Provided that you aren't diabetic, your body will produce a hormone called insulin to regulate this increase in blood sugar level. Your body needs to keep its blood sugar level within a normal range of 90 to 120 mg/dl.

When your body releases insulin in response to blood sugar ingestion, it often over-regulates the blood sugar, driving it below the normal range. This low sugar level then causes a sugar craving. Consequently, you may feel the need to eat additional sources of sugar to satisfy this internal condition.

This additional sugar will again spike blood sugar and cause the release of more insulin. So you will crave even more sugar! This cycle explains the "sweet tooth" you may experience after dinner. A "sweet tooth" isn't genetic, and isn't something that is only germane to you or your family. It's the craving of sugar due to the insulin response, an addictive cycle from which most people cannot break free. This is exactly why many Americans accumulate fat and become obese.

Glucagon is another important hormone; however, it works in an inverse relationship to insulin. When the body produces insulin, it can't produce glucagon. The detrimental aspect here is that glucagon is one of the hormones that helps burn and oxidize fat. Therefore, whenever you eat sugar your body goes through the insulin response cycle. The body is then prevented from producing glucagon and burning fat. Thus, *you cannot burn fat when you are consuming most sugars.* You're trapping fat in your body!

Slow-releasing complex carbohydrates, such as brown rice and sweet potatoes, do not cause *as*

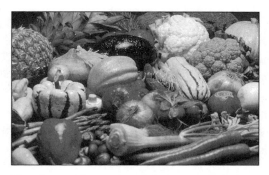

Though vegetables contain carbohydrates, most don't dramatically elevate blood sugar levels. Vegetables are essential and should be consumed at least twice daily.

quick a change in the blood sugar level compared to simple fast-releasing carbohydrates. Thus the body does not need as much insulin as quickly to regulate the blood sugar level. Most fast sugar releasing complex carbohydrates cause a dramatic spike in blood sugar and more insulin is required to regulate it. These foods include most enriched white complex carbohydrates such as white bread, bagels, dough, white pasta, white rice, pretzels, white crackers and white potatoes. Fast sugar releasing complex carbohydrates cause a similar response in your blood sugar as simple carbohydrates (sugar) such as table sugar, fruit, candy and honey.

Fast-releasing complex carbohydrates are not supportive of stabilizing blood sugar levels and reducing your body fat. However, whether fast- or slow-releasing, it is important not to consume too much of any kind of carbohydrate. This is because a large quantity of any carbohydrate will cause an insulin response.

A growing health problem in this country is type two diabetes, also known as adult onset diabetes. The development of this condition is due in part to poor nutritional habits, inadequate exercise and increasing body fat. The American Diabetes Association, in its 1999 Annual Report, states that type two diabetes is "a metabolic disorder resulting from the body's inability to make enough, or properly use, insulin. It is the most common form of the disease. Type two diabetes accounts for ninety to ninety-five percent of diabetes. Type two diabetes is nearing epidemic proportions, due to an increased number of older Americans and a greater prevalence of obesity and sedentary lifestyles." Through the reduction of body fat, eating supportive meals frequently, and developing lean muscle tissue, you may greatly decrease your chances of developing type two diabetes.

Food Chart of Sugar

Simple sugars (carbohydrates): Awful for losing body fat. They spike blood sugar levels, elevate insulin, and should only be consumed on cheat days.

- Table sugar
- Candy
- Fruit
- Fructose
- High fructose corn syrup
- Honey
- Soda pop

Fast-releasing complex carbohydrates: Detrimental to losing body fat. They spike blood sugar levels, elevate insulin, and should only be consumed on cheat days.

- White bread
- White pasta
- Enriched wheat bread
- White or enriched rice
- Crackers
- Bagels
- Pizza
- Pretzels
- White potatoes
- Carrots
- Corn (whole corn, on the cob, popcorn, corn tortillas)
- Any bread or dough-based starch

Slow-releasing carbohydrates: In moderation, they help reduce body fat, stabilize blood sugar levels, and stabilize insulin. Provide a good energy source.

- 100% wheat bread
- 100% wheat pasta
- Sweet potatoes
- Yams
- Whole grain oatmeal
- Brown rice
- 100% whole grain couscous

If a product doesn't say "sugar" in the ingredients list, it doesn't mean that it's sugar-free. Sugar comes in many forms. If you read food labels, be on the lookout for the following ingredients.

Various Types of Simple Sugars

Glucose	Fructose
Corn syrup	Barley malt
Glycerin	Maltose
Honey	Sucrose
Fruit extracts	Dextrin
Cellulose	Lactose
Levulose	Aorbitol
Xylitol	Mannitol

The items listed above are all examples of simple sugars. Marketers love to hide these sugars in the ingredients list. However, if you read the ingredients list and know some of their tricks, you'll be less apt to be fooled by these sneaky devils.

Many Americans have a growing concern about using artificial sweeteners. When artificial sweeteners are substituted for sugar, your body will be able to reduce its body fat more efficiently and forego the insulin response cycle. Over time, this may reduce your chance of developing obesity and/or type two diabetes. As far as the safety of using artificial sweeteners, I believe they are safe when used in moderation. In their 1999 Annual Report, the American Diabetes Association approved the use of three artificial sweeteners in moderate amounts: saccharin, aspartame and acesulfame potassium. I tell my clients to use diet drinks and artificial sweeteners instead of sugar-based drinks or sugar.

The Biggest Offender

I guarantee if you're not looking out for your own health and fitness, no one else will. Don't count on the government, USDA, FDA or any other agency to protect you from deceitful marketers or from themselves! In June 2002, President George W. Bush signed a $190 billion farm bill that included a ten-year $4 billion program that will pay farmers to grow corn. You may be asking yourself, "What is wrong with growing corn?" The problem is, we struggle to get rid of the surplus of corn we already produce. The average bushel of corn (fifty-six pounds) sells for about $2, but it cost farmers more than $3 to grow it!

The government is not currently designing a program that encourages farmers to plant less corn, which would decrease the supply and raise the price. This way, farmers could make a profit and tax dollars would not have to subsidize production. Instead, the government subsidizes and guarantees 125,000 square miles of corn (double the size of New York State) to be produced each year. Now I am not leading you on an economic treatise on farming and showing you how the government is wasting your tax dollars. Rather, I am demonstrating to you how over-production of corn is impacting your health and fitness.

Corn surplus is turned into feed, sugar by-products, and plastics. Many cattle and chicken farmers now give their animals corn feed to fatten them because, thanks to governmental subsidies, it is the cheapest food you can give an animal. The problem is that most of these animals have evolved to eat grass. A corn diet creates havoc in their digestive systems, making it necessary to give them antibiotics to prevent illness and infections. Corn-fed chicken, meat and even fish are a lesser source of protein and not as nutritious as naturally raised animals.

Now remember, corn is a natural filler that fattens hogs, pigs and humans. In fact, if a client tells me they ate corn, I ask them if they enjoy eating like a hog! It sounds silly, but it gets my point across. Even worse than the abundance of corn consumed on the cob, frozen, through corn-fed animals and processed cereal is the abomination of high fructose corn syrup.

High fructose corn syrup is found in everything from soda pop to Snackwell cookies to Weight Watchers nutrition bars. Many manufacturers switched from sugar to high fructose corn syrup in the 1980s because it was inexpensive. It is estimated that nearly ten percent of all calories an adult consumes come from corn sweeteners and nearly twenty percent for children. If you think you're not eating high fructose corn syrup, look at the ingredients list of some of your favorite foods, such as cereal, chips, muffins, bread, cookies, crackers, soda pop, nutrition bars, bagels and PopTarts, to name a few.

With the increase in the prevalence of corn and high fructose corn syrup, it is no surprise that the United States has reached epidemic levels in obesity and type two diabetes. both of which are highly preventable. Michael Pollan, author of *The Botany of Desire: A Plant's Eye View of the World*, adds this about the consequences of high fructose corn syrup found as a sweetener in so many products: "This would be bad enough for the American waistline, but there's also preliminary research suggesting that high fructose corn syrup is metabolized differently than other sugars, making it potentially more harmful." He further states, "A recent study at the University of Minnesota found that a diet high in fructose (as compared to glucose) elevates triglyceride levels in men shortly after eating, a phenomenon that has been linked to an increased risk of obesity and heart disease."

If you want to lose body fat and prevent diabetes and obesity, stay away from corn and especially high fructose corn syrup. Always check the ingredients of foods you or your children eat.

Alcohol

My clients often want to know what effect alcohol has on gaining or losing body fat. Alcohol, whether it's beer, wine or hard liquor, is comprised of alcohol and sugar. Both of these ingredients will significantly affect your blood sugar and insulin, and thus your body fat will increase.

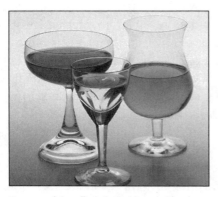

In the *Quebec Family Study*, alcohol intake was associated with a high daily caloric intake and fat gain, particularly in the trunk area. Tremblay and Cigolini, in their paper, "Body fatness in active individuals reporting low lipid and alcohol intake," reported the finding of "a positive association between usual alcohol ingestion and body fat accumulation at the trunk." I usually tell my clients they are free to consume up to two servings of alcohol a week. Any more than two drinks a week will make the reduction of body fat difficult. A lot of alcohol consumption will make you downright fat! Please drink sparingly.

Because of the effect alcohol has on blood sugar, it is important to limit your consumption to two drinks per week.

Fruit

A concept many of my clients have a hard time understanding is the adverse consequences of consuming fruit. You've been told for most of your life that any type of fruit is good to eat at any time. Also, you've heard if you eat a lot of fruit and lay off junk food, you will lose weight. I want you to be aware that fruit is sugar! Fructose, or fruit sugar, reacts in the body with insulin and glucagon just like sucrose, honey, or table sugar, so your body can't differentiate between the sugar in an apple and the sugar in a Snickers bar! In fact, the amount of sugar contained in a banana is equivalent to two and a half Snickers bars!

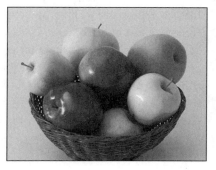

Remember, fruit is sugar and consumption yields an insulin response, which can increase your body fat.

I'm not saying that you can never eat fruit. What I am saying is that you should know that the consumption of fruit will affect your blood sugar levels and insulin secretion. I know what the FDA suggests in the food pyramid. But maybe, in all the FDA's infinite wisdom, it doesn't work. The food pyramid was never intended to help people reduce body fat. In fact, many progressive and intelligent physicians have been trying to change the food pyramid for years by lowering the amount of carbohydrates suggested. However, the FDA and Congress are slow to change. You will hear more about the new food pyramid in the next few years.

I am not suggesting that candy and fruit contain the same amounts of vitamins and minerals. But remember, vegetables contain more vitamins and minerals than fruit, and you are now eating them twice a day. Sugar from fruit is as addictive as sugar from candy or white bread, and the consumption of it makes it very difficult to lower your body fat. I typically reserve eating fruit for my cheat day. So if your goal is to lose fat and inches, eat fruit sparingly.

Break yourself free from sugar!

If you are a bit of a sugarholic—and most of us are from time to time—you need to do something that is going to be difficult. You need to give up sugar for three days, eat the way I recommend and exercise. If you do these things, your sugar cravings will diminish. The first day will be somewhat uncomfortable, since your body is conditioned to having excess sugar in its system.

The second day will be even more challenging and you could even get a headache, and the third day will be the most difficult. You may want to break down and give into the craving, but hold fast. The end is near! By the fourth day you will no longer crave sugars. You will have broken free from the physical addiction.

Now, I'm not saying that you'll never desire chocolate chip cookies or ice cream again. I don't believe that you should ever give up anything you enjoy forever. However, you'll notice a change in your tastes and appetite. You'll begin to desire foods such as brown rice and green vegetables (hard to believe, but true!), and you'll soon enjoy good lean sources of protein. Believe it or not, you'll learn to listen to your body and nourish it with foods that will support your goals.

Sugar warning!

SUMMARY

- Sugar causes an insulin response that ultimately leads to fat gain.

- Always check the ingredients list of foods so that you are less likely to be deceived by slick marketers.

- Be aware of corn and high fructose corn syrup. They both contain an excess amount of sugar.

- Consume no more than two servings of alcohol per week.

- Fruit is a simple sugar, so limit your consumption.

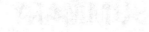

8

DON'T BE FOOLED
BY SLICK MARKETERS

Daryl, the duped

Daryl came to me as a last hope. He had tried all of the weight loss programs before; in fact, he told me that his attempts included weight loss centers, low protein diets, low fat diets, cabbage soup diets, frivolous home fitness equipment, aerobic classes, health club memberships, over-the-counter metabolism-increasing pills, and prescription fat blockers. He also attempted to eat "fat free," "low fat" and "reduced fat." He only bought foods that were "natural," "lean" and "light."

After listening to Daryl share for half an hour what he had tried to lose weight and shape and tone his body, I was dizzy! Simultaneously, I felt sympathy for him. It wasn't his fault he was out of shape. He tried very hard to take control of his body and health, but by listening to bad advice. Unfortunately, he'll *never* get into shape following this ineffective information. He, as well as millions of other individuals, have been misinformed and deceived by marketers. Misinformation and deception in the health and fitness industry is the main reason why I developed this system and wrote this book.

After listening to Daryl's sad but common story, I began to educate him on why his attempts hadn't been successful. I said, "Daryl, you didn't fail. You've been deceived into trying what you wanted to believe!" Products are manufactured and marketed to sell and make money. Consequently, there is widespread deception in this industry.

I informed Daryl that he would only need three things to get into the best shape and health of his life: weight training, eating supportive meals frequently and performing cardiovascular training in moderation. I told him to forget about everything else he thought he knew about losing fat and scale weight. I said, "Unlike what marketers boast, it isn't quick, it isn't easy and it doesn't work 'like magic'! There's no special exercise machine that burns fat quicker, and there are no magic metabolism increasing pills. Diets don't work long-term and food manufacturers want to sell their fat free and low fat products."

Daryl stopped me and said, "I understand how I've been deceived with exercise machines and magic pills, but I'm not sure that food manufacturers can legally mislead the public with regards to their products." Daryl's comment was good. How can food manufacturers legally deceive and misinform the public?

I explained to him that food manufacturers want their products to sell. Since most people want to eat well, a product that claims to be fat free sounds more appealing than a product that doesn't. Food manufacturers know this and use loopholes in the labeling laws to market their products. The most common loophole has to do with serving sizes. For example, a product can be labeled fat free if it has less than .5 grams of fat per serving. Food manufacturers can get any product to be less than .5 grams per serving if they make the serving size small enough. Check the serving size of fat free cooking oil or low fat cookies. You may be surprised!

I also warned Daryl that, just because a product is labeled fat free, it doesn't mean it's supportive of your goals to lose fat and scale weight. It's important to know that dietary fat and body fat are two separate things. You can gain or lose body fat independently of eating fat free, low fat or reduced fat. In fact, most fat free products contain very high portions of sugar to give them a better taste. Fat free cookies are an excellent example of high concentrations of sugar or high fructose corn syrup added to replace fat in the product.

I instructed Daryl to disregard food label hype. I told him to read the ingredients list on the back of the package and discover what is truly in the product. If a product is high in sugar, it won't be supportive of your goals. If a product has a tiny serving size, it's important not to overuse the product because it will be high in calories. Always read the ingredients and serving size. They'll reveal the contents of the product.

Don't be fooled by slick marketers

Food manufacturers know one thing: how to make money by selling food. The words they put on their labels entice you to purchase their product, for example, "Light," "Low Fat," "Fat Free," "Reduced Fat," "Lean" and "Healthy." However, these foods might not resemble anything close to what I categorized earlier as supportive. Don't let the slick product marketers fool you into believing you are purchasing a product that will help you improve your health and fitness. I'll teach you some tips to help avoid being seduced by these tricky manufacturers.

First, when you shop for food, I suggest that you limit your purchases to the perimeter of the store. This is where you will find staple items such as meat, fish, eggs, poultry and vegetables. This suggestion alone will save you hundreds of dollars each year on deceitful, misleading and wrongly labeled garbage. You will not only save money, you'll also save time and extra inches on your waistline.

Next, it's important to have a grocery list already prepared before you start shopping (see Chapter 17). If a food isn't on the list, don't buy it. If a food wasn't important or supportive to you when you prepared the list, it still isn't important or supportive when you see the bright colorful packaging and deceptive label. Don't buy it!

How do food manufacturers get away with their deceptive claims? Let's take a closer look.

"Fat Free"

Many food labels have the words "fat free" plastered all over their packaging—for one reason only. Those words *sell products.* In fact, I read a report in the *New England Journal of Medicine* that states that each year, food manufacturers produce over 50,000 new products claiming to be fat free, low fat, reduced fat or light. Does the label accurately represent what ingredients are in the product? In far too many cases, absolutely not. The label has little to do with the ingredients or quality of the food being sold, but it has everything to do with the bottom line and increased profits. Do you really think that food manufacturers are looking out for your best interest or theirs?

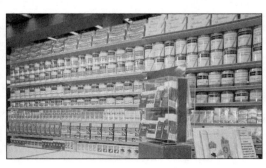

You'll find out if you go to the grocery store, or perhaps only as far as your refrigerator, and look at one of the "fat free" butter substitutes. Look at the ingredients.

Hundreds of new low fat products are introduced into stores each years.

You will likely find the main ingredient is hydrogenated oil. Hydrogenated oils are pure fat! So how do the labelers get away with calling a product that is pure fat, fat free? Labeling laws have been created with massive loopholes that allow food manufacturers to mislead or, in some cases, blatantly lie about their products. The loophole usually involves the serving size. If a product has less than .5 grams of fat *per serving*, the product can legally be labeled fat free. How do you think that food manufacturers can get any product to have less than .5 grams of fat per serving? The answer is by decreasing the serving size under .5 grams! The law doesn't define how small a serving size can be. Consequently, manufacturers can label all their products fat free if their serving size is small enough.

This is seen most clearly in sprayed cooking oil. Cooking oil, or any oil for that matter, is by definition 100 percent fat. However, many manufacturers of cooking oil label their products as fat free. If you look at the serving size, you will discover that the suggested serving size is a one-third-second spray!

I've tried many times, and maybe you're better than me, but I can't hold the nozzle one-third of a second. I either get nothing out or the spray lasts at least one second. If the spray is one second, I'm consuming three serving sizes according to the manufacturer. Some clients tell me they hold their spray long enough to coat the pan. In my estimation, that's at least three seconds. Three seconds of spray is nine servings! Also, the manufacturer claims that there are 550 servings per container. I defy anyone to get 550 equal servings out of that aerosol container.

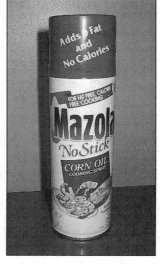

Look at the serving size of products.

"95 Percent Fat Free"

This has always been one of my favorites. If you were to eat a stick of butter (please don't do it!), you would be consuming 100 percent of your calories from fat. If you were to take the same stick of butter and mix it with water and then drink the solution, you would still be getting 100 percent of your calories from fat, since water doesn't contain any calories.

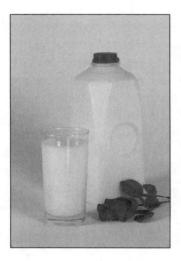

Manufacturers add water to reduce the fat in milk.

If you were a food manufacturer and you wanted to sell your butter/water solution to health-conscious consumers, you wouldn't sell much if you put the words "100 percent of calories from fat" on the label. However, you could be a little tricky and modify the solution to have the same amount of butter and water by *volume*, not by calories. You could then label your product as fifty percent fat free by volume. Even though 100 percent of the calories is still from fat, the law doesn't stipulate that you cannot label by volume. If fifty percent fat free doesn't sound good enough, no problem! More water can be added to get whatever percentage you desire, such as ninety-five percent fat free. Now that sounds more appealing, doesn't it?

And don't think that only butter is manipulated. Meats and poultry are also commonly pumped with water to reduce the fat by volume on the label. However, the biggest target for years has been milk. Milk is mostly water and 100 percent of the calories come from fat. You commonly see milk labeled as skim (no fat), one percent fat, two percent fat or whole (which they claim is five percent fat). The only difference in any milk product is the amount of water that is added. Skim milk has the most water added, thus, it is nearly fat free by volume. However, don't be deceived. No type of milk has less than forty percent of its calories from fat! It's deceptive, but it sells.

Before you get all worked up about the fact the food industry has been lying to you for years—and, by the way, let me tell you it has—you can't possibly fight against them. There's too much money involved. Senators and congressmen are given billions of dollars each year by political action coalitions and lobbyists, such as food manufacturers, to ensure the laws don't change.

I suggest you educate yourself instead of fighting the food industry. You can't save the nation, but you can educate yourself and your family. It is crucial to know how food manufacturers manipulate product labels. Don't let yourself be deceived by their slick marketing strategies. This knowledge will help you immensely in improving your health and fitness.

So how do you see through the deceptive labeling?

On any food label, manufacturers are required to list ingredients in *descending order of abundance*. If any item in that list includes fat (oil, lard, butter, whole milk, etc.), you can't be looking at a fat free product, regardless of what the marketers claim in big print on the package.

Manufacturers are also required to list the number of calories per serving and the number of calories from fat, protein and carbohydrates. First, find the serving size on the label and make sure it's more than .5 grams. Then *ignore* the section providing percentage of daily value because it refers to what the government believes the percentage breakdown would be of proteins, carbohydrates and fats based on a 2,000 calorie a day diet. Who said anything about 2,000 calories a day? And how does the government know what our nutritional goals are?

Nutrition Facts

Serving size: 1/2 cup
Servings per container: 2

Amount Per Serving

Calories 180	Calories from Fat 90
	% Daily Value
Total fat 10g	**15%**
Saturated Fat 4g	**20%**
Cholesterol 0mg	**0%**
Sodium 0mg	**0%**
Total Carbohydrates 10.5g	**4%**
Sugars 2g	
Protein 12g	

Summary of percentage of fat by calories

- Product contains 10g of fat per serving and 180 calories per serving.
- Each gram of fat contains nine calories.
- Calories of fat per serving = 10 x 9 = 90.
- Percentage of fat per serving is 180/90 = .5 or 50 percent.

Divide the number of calories from fat by the total number of calories per serving to determine what percentage of the food is fat. For example, if a label indicates that the food contains 100 calories per serving, and thirty calories are from fat, it is easy to see that the food is thirty percent fat. The same calculations can be done for carbohydrates and protein.

You can also use the grams per serving to determine the percentage of calories contained in a product. You've already learned that each gram of fat contains nine calories and protein and carbohydrates contain four calories per gram. So, if a product has ten grams of fat per serving, multiply ten by nine and you will get ninety. That equals ninety calories of fat per serving. If the total number of calories per serving were 180, then ninety divided by 180 would be .5 or fifty percent fat.

I would suggest for any product that it is important to keep overall fat intake down to twenty-five to thirty percent per serving unless the product is an essential fatty acid. If a product is more than thirty percent fat by serving, it can be harmful to the body and to your fitness results because of the high caloric density.

"Sugar Free"

By now I hope you're becoming much less trusting of labels. By knowing the tricks of food manufacturers and how the labeling laws work or better yet, don't work, you're learning how to protect yourself. As many of my clients know, the gross over-consumption of sugar is one of the biggest reasons why people get fat.

Being from Buffalo, New York—birthplace of the Buffalo chicken wing and home to *long* winters—I see "fatness" or, to use the medical term, "adiposity" every day. I see obese, overweight and out-of-shape people everywhere. They're typically drinking a soda (not a diet soda!), orange juice or, better yet, a beer! They may be eating bagels, pretzels, pizza, popcorn or some other type of enriched starchy white carbohydrate. And this phenomenon isn't isolated to just Buffalo. I was recently in South Beach and Miami and you would be shocked to see all of the fat and out of shape bodies soaking in the South Florida sun. Additionally, if you believe that your body fat is above acceptable levels, I want you to seriously reconsider your choice of wearing spandex, belly shirts or tank tops!

Let me re-emphasize—if you consume more than a moderate amount of sugar, you will gain body fat. To give you some specific examples, a twenty-ounce bottle of Coke contains 100 calories per serving and two and a half servings per container. So if you drink the entire container (which isn't that hard to do), you'll consume 250 calories. Coke contains

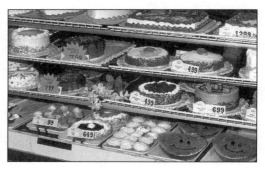

Watch out for products that contain large amounts of sugar.

69

twenty-seven grams of sugar per serving. Now remember, there are two and a half servings per container, so that equals 67.5 grams of sugar for a twenty-ounce bottle of Coke.

Maybe you didn't know this, but one teaspoon of sugar is equivalent to four grams. So if you divide 67.5 grams by four grams per teaspoon, the twenty-ounce bottle of Coke contains almost seventeen teaspoons of sugar! Most of us would never dream of sitting in front of the sugar bowl and eating seventeen straight teaspoons of sugar. It would be awful! Sickening! However, many of us would not hesitate to consume one if not more Coca-Colas per day. It's no wonder, then, sixty-one percent of Americans are defined as overweight.

You might be thinking to yourself, "Well, that's soda pop. I never drink soda." If you don't drink soda, good. Soda won't do anything to support your muscle and it will create havoc with your insulin response. You will also gain body fat. However, soda pop is not the only product that contains a deceptive amount of sugar.

Let's take a look at orange juice. A common brand of orange juice contains 120 calories per serving and two servings per sixteen-ounce bottle. Therefore, the entire sixteen ounces of juice contains 240 calories. Also, this bottle of orange juice contains thirty-one grams of sugar per serving or sixty-one grams total. Once again, if you divide sixty-one grams of sugar by four teaspoons per gram, you get 15.25 teaspoons in the bottle of juice! Since the juice has 15.25 teaspoons of sugar per sixteen-ounce bottle and Coke has 17 teaspoons per twenty-ounce bottle, the juice contains *more sugar per ounce* than Coke! As I mentioned before, if you want to lose fat, you must carefully examine the labels of products you consume.

	Coke	Orange Juice
Size in ounces	20	16
Calories	250	240
Grams of sugar	67.5	61
Teaspoons of sugar	17	15.25
Teaspoons of sugar per ounce	.85	.95

I've seen packages with labels that indicate that the enclosed brownies are "sugar free," yet the most prominent ingredient is fructose. Sure, it's fruit sugar and marketers can call it natural; however, it's still sugar. Remember that simple sugars include glucose, fructose, corn syrup, barley malt, glycerin, glycerol, honey, sucrose, and fruit extracts. It's in your best interest to avoid (or at least limit) consumption.

Don't be fooled by slick marketers

SUMMARY

- Look at product labels to see if manufacturers are "sneaking" fats and sugars into the ingredients list.

- Remember, food manufacturers' intention is to persuade you to purchase their product, sometimes with less than honest claims.

- Consuming too much sugar or fat will increase your body fat and jeopardize your health and fitness goals.

9

AEROBIC EXERCISE CAN MAKE YOU FATTER

Mary, the aerobic freak

Mary arranged a consultation with me about losing weight and toning her body. She was somewhat different than many people with whom I typically consult. She wasn't a novice exerciser and had attended various health clubs for years. She knew the importance of exercise for both her health and fitness. I said to Mary, "I understand that you've been exercising for years. In what ways would you like me to help you?" As she grabbed her butt, Mary responded, "I want to know exactly what I have to do to tone my body and lose *this*!"

I asked her what exercise she had been doing. She told me that she had been doing one hour of cardiovascular training every Monday, Wednesday, and Friday on either the treadmill or the stair stepper. On Tuesdays, Thursdays and Saturdays she attended step aerobic classes that lasted about ninety minutes. Before I could respond, she blurted out, "Do you think that I should increase my cardio time on Mondays, Wednesdays and Fridays, or should I do additional cardio on Sunday?"

I calmly asked her, "Do you want to get a fatter fanny?" Mary was shocked and said, "What do you mean?" I proceeded to explain to her that she was constantly breaking down her muscle tissue. This woman was doing seven and a half hours of cardiovascular training a week! The huge amount of cardio was burning her muscle as energy. I explained to her that the less muscle tissue she has on her body, the fewer calories and fat she will burn. Further, I tried to impress upon her the fact she was actually *slowing down* her metabolism by doing so much cardiovascular training.

Many exercisers are similar to Mary and inaccurately believe that more exercise is better. If spending twenty-five minutes doing aerobic training is good, forty-five minutes must be better. Some misinformed people also think, "I want to get into the best shape as quickly as I can, so I'll do sixty minutes of aerobic training every day." I urge you not to fall victim to this misconception. I'll repeat again: it is *essential*, in order to speed your metabolism and lower your body fat, that you don't exercise away your muscle tissue by doing *too much* cardiovascular training!

Aerobic exercise can make you fatter

What if you're really committed to getting into better shape? Let's say that you're absolutely dedicated to dropping fat and "sweating off" the weight. You're faithfully walking forty minutes on the treadmill and performing aerobic step class four to five days a week. You're really trying hard and doing everything in your power to finally get in shape. How do you think you would you feel at the end of a month if you were actually fatter than before you started this difficult exercise program? I think that you'd feel cheated and angry. I believe that you might never go to the gym again. You might feel that exercise doesn't work and isn't right for you. In this chapter, I will explain how cardiovascular exercise can make you fatter and how my system will prevent you from ever having this happen.

Cardiovascular and aerobic exercises are the same and I will uses these terms interchangeably throughout this book. The question is, how can increased cardiovascular exercise make you fatter? Please stay with me while I try to simplify this as much as possible.

When you eat complex carbohydrates, they're slowly converted into glucose and stored in the muscle as glycogen, which is a fuel reserve for your muscles. Glycogen stores are limited, so if you don't eat sufficiently to keep those stores full, your aerobic session may exhaust your stored sugar. If this happens, your body will tap into muscle to create its own fuel by converting some amino acids (the building blocks of muscle and protein) into sugars that can provide the fuel needed for body functions.

The only way your body can access those amino acids is to break down muscle tissue. Thus it is possible during aerobic exercise to exercise away precious muscle tissue. By now, you understand that this will have a long-term negative effect, making your body more efficient at storing fat!

I am *not* suggesting that you don't perform aerobic exercise. In fact, in Lose Fat Forever I recommend you include aerobic exercise several times per week. However, it's vital to perform aerobic exercise in moderation. The specific amount of time you spend doing aerobic exercise actually depends upon your physical condition, the amount of muscle you have and your fitness goals.

For example, if you've been lifting weights, have good mus-

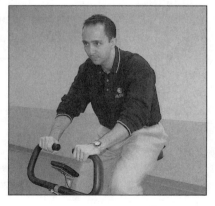

Maintain your lean muscle tissue by performing aerobic training in moderation.

cle tone and low body fat, you should probably never exceed fifteen to twenty minutes of aerobic activity at one time in order to preserve your lean muscle tissue. On the other hand, if you're relatively new to weight training, have limited muscle tone and body fat above eighteen percent for men and twenty percent for women, you could probably perform up to thirty to thirty-five minutes of aerobic exercise per session without breaking down a significant amount of your lean muscle tissue.

The exact amount of desirable aerobic training varies on an individual basis according to the factors previously mentioned. If you aren't sure whether you're performing too much or too little aerobic training, contact a personal fitness professional for assistance.

For those of you who belong to a health club or have ever been in a health club before, I want you to visualize people exercising. You can probably recollect that the majority of the people exercising were performing cardiovascular exercise. The stair steppers were full, the elliptical climbers were humming and there was probably even a line and sign-up sheet to use the treadmills. If you can picture the people using this equipment, were most of them lean and toned or soft and flabby? I've found most of them to have higher amounts of body fat and many were significantly out-of-shape or obese.

Now I want you to visualize the people who were using the free weights. Probably less than ten percent of the people in the gym were in this area. Younger men, some women and a few determined individuals working with a personal trainer mostly inhabit this area. Were most of the people in the free weight area lean and toned or soft and flabby? I've found, and I'm sure you'll agree, the majority of them are lean and toned. They have developed lean muscle tissue and generally appear to be in good shape.

Do you want to work out like people who are soft and flabby or lean and toned? I know you want "less jiggle and more ripple." So work out with free weights and perform a limited amount of cardiovascular training.

Anytime you perform aerobic activities, your body has three options for fuel. It can burn blood sugar, fat or muscle. If your blood sugar is fluctuating due to going long periods without supportive nutrition, your body will release less fat. If you consume simple sugars, fat release will be compromised due to insulin production. If you don't take in enough calories to support your activity, your body will actually "cling" to fat and will cause aerobic movement to seek out sugar as a fuel source. And, if you perform aerobic exercise for a prolonged period of time, your body will seek out the slowest and most abundant energy source, which, consequently, is your muscles. Thus aerobic exercise may *not* utilize your stored body fat at all. *It may make you fatter!*

In Part III: Body in Motion, which includes the workout sections, you will clearly see the relationship between your time spent with weight training and cardiovascular training. On three days per week, I provide you with exact weight training exercises that will take you approximately thirty to forty minutes to perform. I also provide you with precise information regarding a moderate amount of cardiovascular training six days a week. Don't worry. These workouts are within your capabilities and will maintain your interest. Remember, you now have the information and desire to succeed.

Aerobic exercise can make you fatter

SUMMARY

- Perform cardiovascular training in moderation.

- Performing too much cardiovascular training may break down your muscle tissue. This will slow down your metabolism and make you fatter.

- Spend less time doing cardiovascular training and more time engaging in weight training.

- Contact a personal fitness professional if you have questions regarding weight training or cardiovascular training workouts.

10

SPEND LESS TIME IN THE GYM

Mary, the aerobic freak, part two

Returning to the discussion in the last chapter about Mary, I recommended that she perform cardiovascular training no more than three times per week for thirty minutes at a time. I also told her that she needed to do weight training three times a week and eat in a supportive manner. Mary's biggest concern was the concept of spending less time on the treadmill while attaining better results. She didn't believe it was possible to look better and lose more fat doing one and a half hours of cardiovascular training instead of seven and a half hours a week.

As you can imagine, this conversation was not as straightforward as I just described. The consultation took nearly ninety minutes. At the end of the consultation, she was still not completely convinced my recommendations would work.

I don't blame her. She was previously led to believe that the more cardiovascular training she performed, the more calories and fat she would burn. Mary was watching the calorie counter on the treadmill and equating it to the number of calories she believed she consumed in a day. By the way, the calorie counter on cardiovascular machines is just a gauge,

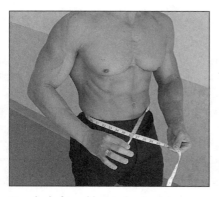

Drop body fat and lose inches by doing aerobic training in moderation and spending less time in the gym.

something that equipment manufacturers have included on the machinery as a feature to occupy you. It doesn't accurately measure your caloric output, so don't be concerned with it.

I finally convinced Mary to try the program for a few months. I promised her that after two months of training with weights, doing less cardiovascular training and eating supportive meals frequently, she would dramatically reduce her body fat. In fact, I bet my reputation on it.

In just two months of training with me, she reduced her body fat 4.5 percent and dropped two inches around her waist and hips! Incidentally, she lost eleven pounds of scale weight, but I want to re-emphasize that scale weight means nothing. Mary had lost scale weight dozens of times before, but she never lowered her body fat and increased her metabolism. The reduction of scale weight is a byproduct of low body fat, but remember, it isn't the most critical issue. More importantly, she told me that, finally, her "a-- looked great in jeans!" She was thrilled. She found out how she could spend less time in the gym and get better results.

Spend less time in the gym

You're a busy person. I'm sure you have many career and personal commitments that keep you busy every day. You most likely can't afford to spend hours each day at the gym, hoping to get into better shape. Well, the good news is that you don't have to! Lose Fat Forever is designed to maximize the time you spend exercising each day so you can attain the health and fitness you desire and still have time to focus on other important facets of your life.

Life isn't particularly enjoyable when you no longer fit into your clothes and when you feel tired throughout the day. When you have a negative self-image, and when you have to limit activities you would like to do, such as mountain bike riding, roller-blading and hiking through the wilderness. The quality of your life will be compromised.

Your health and fitness enable you to enjoy all the wonderful aspects of your life. I don't want you to think that you have to give up anything meaningful in your life to attain better health and fitness. When your health and fitness improves, everything becomes more enjoyable. You can do all the activities you've always wanted to do but were afraid to or not able to do for the reasons I previously listed. As I mentioned in the beginning of the book, all the time you need to commit to is three hours or 1.6 percent of the entire week. Is that too much time to dedicate to improve the quality and duration of your life? Now is the time to start living!

Spend less time in the gym

SUMMARY

- Use the Lose Fat Forever system to make your workouts more efficient. Spend less of your valuable time at the gym.

- Increasing your health and fitness enables you to enjoy a more satisfying lifestyle.

- Better health and fitness will enable you to experience all the activities you have always wanted to do.

11

CONTINUING THE SAME WORKOUT WILL RESULT IN— NOTHING!

Jim, the burnout

Jim called me for a consultation because he had heard from colleagues that I was helping people get into wonderful shape. Jim was a small business owner and, like many, he didn't live an active lifestyle. He was six feet tall and weighed 230 pounds. Jim's main goal was to feel better and look like he did when he was in college. Jim wanted to reduce his thirty-eight inch waist to thirty-four inches and be around 200 pounds of lean muscle tone.

Jim started off by stating, "Other fitness instructors had me lifting weights in the past and it didn't work. I got a little stronger, but I didn't get any leaner. Weight training is too monotonous and I'm burned out on weights." I was shocked. I knew from my experiences with hundreds of clients that weight training absolutely works. In fact, weight training is the only way to lose body fat and increase the metabolism permanently. I needed to know what Jim tried that did not work.

I asked him to describe his previous weight training routine. Jim said, "I would do a weight training circuit designed by a fitness instructor three times a week. It was a series of weight-bearing machines, probably around ten different ones, both upper body and lower body." I asked how many times he went through the circuit and he said twice each workout. I then asked him what else he did with weights and he said, "That's it."

I asked if the circuit or exercises ever changed and Jim said, "No. The instructor told me those ten machines hit all the major muscle groups." I asked him if he ever varied the weight or resistance of the machines and he said, "No." Then I asked Jim if he ever lifted free weights and once again the answer was "No." I finally asked Jim how long he had done that particular circuit and he said, "About eight weeks, then I just quit." I replied, "You know, you're right. If you do the same exercises with the same weights and in the same order three times a week you'll burn out and not get any results."

Jim looked confused and seemed a little bit stunned. I told him the circuit training he had performed was good for the first week of the program, but the circuit routine, the exercises and the resistance must change. I explained how muscle tissue is adaptive. If you don't constantly change the load or stimuli to the muscle, the muscle tissue won't have to adapt and change. Therefore, lean muscle tissue can't be developed, body fat won't decrease and results won't be attained. The body will get accustomed to anything done repeatedly.

I told Jim that working with resistance machines is all right, but working with free weights is much better. When you work with free weights, the body *must* stabilize and balance the weight, which utilizes more calories. Also, most people are either right side or left side dominant. Free weight training makes you use both sides equally. These two aspects of weight training challenge the muscle tissue better and produce more heat (burn more calories) than machine training. Boredom is also reduced with weight training because you must focus your attention on the exercise. The weight isn't on guide rods or cables so you have to be attentive. There's no time for boredom.

84

Continuing the Same Workout Will Result in—Nothing!

Jim said, "It sounds like it makes sense, but I don't know." I asked him to give it a try. I promised him that he wouldn't become bored with my system and that he would see wonderful results like his colleagues. Jim said, "All right, let's do it!"

I knew Jim would do well on my system, but he did better than I even imagined. He was a naturally big guy and was able to develop lean muscle quickly. In four months, he had achieved his thirty-four inch waist and his scale weight was a cool 197 pounds! Jim's body fat had dropped by seven percent in three months and he told me, "I feel better than when I was in college!"

Continuing the same workout will result in—nothing!

The body is amazingly adaptive. When it sheds fat due to changes in eating and activity, it is actually adapting to a new stimulus. Therefore, if you continue with the same workout every week, you will hit what exercisers refer to as a plateau. Your workout will no longer be new and your body will no longer have to adapt to a different stimulus. In fact, your body will get so conditioned to the same workout, it will actually *lose muscle tone and burn less fat* because it doesn't have to work as hard to attain the results. You may even get *fatter* during exercise!

In order to prevent the plateau from occurring, it is *essential* to modify and

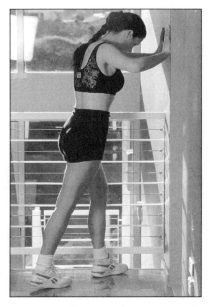

Vary your workouts in order to tone muscle and lose fat.

85

change your workout often. This is where a good personal trainer is valuable. "Periodization" is the term personal trainers use for workout variation. Without getting too scientific, if you constantly change the stimuli to your muscles through work-load, intensity and exercise variation, your body will need to recruit different muscle tissues to meet this new challenge. The Lose Fat Forever system provides the exercise variation that enhances the achievement of your fitness goals.

Because recruitment of different muscle tissue requires your body to perform in a way that is not customary, your mus-cle tissue will be constantly challenged. You will develop lean, toned muscle tissue. I apologize if I lost you here—just remem-ber that lean muscle tissue increases your metabolism and burns body fat. Workout variation is essential to this process. You can't perform the same exercises with the same weights and the same repetitions each workout and expect favorable results.

In the Lose Fat Forever system, our training guidelines include:

- Three weeks of circuit training that involves perform-ing more repetitions with lighter weights.
- Three weeks of endurance training engaging in interval training with shortened rest periods and elevated lactic acid levels.
- Three weeks of power strength training focusing on muscle growth.

If you don't understand the meaning of each of these workouts, don't be concerned at this point. This system will lead you step-by-step through the various exercise programs I have identified. The workouts have been designed to eliminate guesswork on your part; they will tell and show you exactly what exercises to perform, how many repetitions to do and when changes should be made. For additional help, our web-site, www.AlessiFit.com, demonstrates each exercise. Use this website to ensure you are performing them correctly.

If you are reading this book and are still unsure of how to begin the system, I strongly encourage you to schedule an appointment with a personal fitness professional. Even if you don't feel that having a trainer is right for you, a fitness consultation would be useful to get started. A fitness professional can help you define your goals and clarify how this system can help you achieve the success you desire. If you need additional help, contact my office where Don and I can conduct a telephone consultation.

Continuing the same workout will result in—nothing!

SUMMARY

- If you don't change your workout often, you will plateau.

- When you plateau, you will either stay the same or get fatter.

- Following the Lose Fat Forever system will constantly challenge your muscles to adapt to different stimuli by employing workout variation.

- If you are still unsure of how to complete this system, contact a fitness professional or my office for assistance.

12

THERE IS NO SUCH THING AS THE PERFECT TIME!

Dave: "I'll start fresh next week"

This is a story I regret to use as an example, for reasons you will soon understand. Dave was one of the first clients Don and I had worked with. He was in his early forties, overweight and a smoker. He was unathletic and new to exercise, but he wanted to improve his health and fitness. He knew he should take the time to change his unhealthy behaviors and improve his lifestyle.

Dave began his fitness program beautifully. He worked out hard and was beginning to eat better. Within a few weeks he had already lowered his scale weight seven pounds and increased his strength and endurance. He was looking better and, more importantly, feeling better. His body was his first priority.

Unfortunately, after six to eight weeks, Dave began to falter. He worked as a furniture dealer and often had to travel out of town to meet potential buyers. At first, Dave would only miss an occasional workout, but soon this number grew. Within a few months, he was missing workouts regularly. Don and I often spoke to him about recommitting to his body. We asked him, "Dave, you've already made progress and come so far. Do you really want to back track and start all over again?" He responded, "No, I don't want to give up progress, but I'm too busy this week. *I'll start fresh next week.*"

Don and I were new to the fitness business at that time and we believed Dave. We weren't as astute at seeing through excuses as we are now, and we expected him to recommit himself the following week. However, this setback had nothing to do with Dave being overly busy at work. He was making the same excuse millions of individuals do each day—he was procrastinating.

Whenever I hear anybody say, "I'm not going to work out today because I'm too busy" or "I don't feel good today; I'll work out tomorrow," I honestly believe they have good intentions. At the time, they believe they *will* work out later or tomorrow. However, this behavior is a mindset, not a scheduling problem. When you procrastinate or refuse to take action with your body, you're conditioning your mind to neglect your health and fitness. You're sending a mental signal that your body is not your top priority.

This is why it's so important to schedule your workouts and stick to your schedule. No time will ever be perfect and there will never be a better time than now. Another personal trainer and a colleague of mind once told me, "Derek, anyone can work out when they feel good. However, when you work out and don't feel 100 percent or don't have the time, then you'll make progress."

This inconsistent behavior went on for months. Dave put on the seven pounds he had lost plus an additional eight pounds. He lost his strength and his endurance. He felt physically awful and looked terrible, but he kept assuring Don and me that he would *start fresh next week.*

Finally, next week never came. Dave missed his Monday workout appointment. When Don called his house to see why he had missed, he learned that Dave had suffered a heart attack and died at age forty-three. Don and I were shocked.

There is No Such Thing as the Perfect Time!

I'm not telling you this story to scare you. I'm telling you what can happen if you don't make your health and fitness a priority. You, like Dave, are too young and have too much living left to do to allow this ill fate. You will never regret spending time on your body. But do it now—there is no such thing as the perfect time.

There is no such thing as the perfect time!

I've often heard prospective clients tell me the current time isn't good for them to begin a health and fitness program. Some of the most common rationalizations (excuses) I've heard include: "I'm too busy at work," "I have to check my schedule," "I'll begin after the holidays," "I want to wait until the kids are back in school," "I'll be traveling a lot over the next several months," or "I'm busy outdoors in the summer."

I promise if you think long and hard enough you can probably come up with at least five reasons why you *cannot* begin a health and fitness program. In fact, this is exactly what most Americans do. They tell me or themselves why this isn't a good time to begin a healthy lifestyle. Consequently, this is the reason most Americans (sixty-one percent) are overweight or obese. They think everything in their lives must be perfect before they can begin a life improvement system. Unfortunately, no time will ever be perfect! *This is a dangerous mind set that you must avoid!*

You've procrastinated enough and your health and fitness levels have suffered. Every day you procrastinate is another day further from your goals, dreams and better health. Don't make the same mistake that millions of Americans do by convincing yourself that you can't exercise today. The time to do it is now! Even if you're tired; even if you have a mild cough or congestion; even if you have a busy day, do it today! There will never be a better time than now.

There is no such thing as the perfect time!

SUMMARY

- Don't fool yourself into thinking you'll begin to work out tomorrow, next month or after the holidays. Do it now!

- Every day you procrastinate is another day further from your goals, dreams and better health.

- There is no such thing as the perfect time.

13

GET HELP!

Rob, the Type A personality

My personal clientele consists of many successful, assertive and driven men and women. They are captains of industry and leaders of their companies. Their raw energy and focus has enabled them to succeed in the business world—but often to fail miserably in the fitness world. Rob was one of these people.

Rob was fifty-five years old and in rough shape. He was a highly successful financial underwriter but his body was broken down. Rob scheduled a consultation with me and within a few minutes I understood why he needed to achieve better health. He worked in the financial realm, but his passion was flying his own airplane and he was a certified flight instructor. Rob needed to pass a mandatory physical to keep his pilot's certificate and, since he barely passed last year, he was worried.

Rob started off by saying, "Derek, I am fifty-five years old and I cannot see my shoes because of the fat in my stomach. However, my main goal is to lower my blood pressure without medicine, so that I can continue to fly. Now, in the process of achieving this, I wouldn't mind trimming the fat." He further went on to say, "I've been on programs and diets before, and I keep losing and gaining the same twenty pounds. It seems like my attention span is no longer than three months."

Rob's main concern was passing his pilot's physical by lowering his blood pressure. His secondary concern was to lose the fat, but he was worried he could not stick to a program consistently. I asked him, "Have you ever worked with a personal trainer before?" He answered, "Not really. I was given a program and shown around the health club when I joined by one of the salesmen." I then asked him to describe his typical workout. He said, "I started by going to the gym six days a week and performing the exercises I was shown. Then I noticed the exercises other people in the gym were doing and incorporated these exercises into my routine. Every two to three workouts, I tried to add weights or repetitions."

Now I asked Rob the pivotal question, "How do you know whether the others in the gym—the ones you were copying— were doing the right things and performing them properly?" He answered, "Good question. I guess I don't." Further, I asked him if the others shared the same goals he had, to which he answered, "I don't know." I then asked Rob, "When you give flight instructions, do you show the new students around the plane once and then leave them on their own to figure it out themselves or copy off others?" He said, "Of course not. First they need to study flight manuals and pass a written competency exam. Then they need eighty-five assisted hours of flight time with a certified and licensed pilot."

I went on to explain to Rob that the body is like a plane and flight lessons, only much more complex. Modern researchers have spent decades studying the human body and still only know a fraction of the body's intelligence. Most people have little knowledge of anatomy, physiology, kinesiology, cardio-respiratory function and proper weight training techniques. I told Rob, "You would never dream of letting an inexperienced and naive student fly your plane, but with your assertive personality, you jumped right into trying to fly your body without a clue!"

Rob agreed. He then rationalized that he knew more about how a plane or car worked than his own body. In fact, he said, "I have taken better care of both my plane and my car with regular maintenance and service then I have ever taken with my own body!" I told Rob that he is not alone. The problem is that you can buy a new plane or car, but you cannot buy a new body. Like it or hate it, it is the only body you will ever have this time around. So treat it better than all of your worldly possessions, because without it, nothing else matters.

Rob needed help and working with a trainer was the answer for him. He learned how his body worked and how to increase his metabolism permanently. He also felt better knowing he was taking care of himself. He said, "I wish I would have taken the time to work with a trainer and learn about my body years ago." Incidentally, Rob passed his last two pilot's physicals. I cut back his workouts from six days a week to four. He has lost thirty-five pounds of fat and now fits comfortable into size 34 jeans. But best of all, Rob has been working out regularly for the past two years and has incorporated fitness into his lifestyle.

Get help!

In most of life's endeavors, a certain knowledge or competency is needed to perform a function, task or job. For example, a written test and a road test must be passed before you can be a licensed driver. Examinations must be passed satisfactorily before you can be issued college degrees, and certification exams and thesis written for advanced degrees. However, most human beings have no idea how their body works and have never taken classes or spent the time to learn valuable information. Everyone has a body, but it does not come with a user's manual. Unfortunately, most individuals gather information about their health and fitness through mis-leading sources such as infomercials, magazines, television, in-store products and through gossip.

I am not saying that everyone must take classes in anato-my, physiology, kinesiology (the study of movement), nutri-tion and weight training principles, though it would improve their knowledge of their body immensely. Nor am I suggesting that everyone become a certified personal trainer. What I am highly recommending is that if you want to learn how to lose fat, reduce your waistline, lower your blood pressure, live longer, reduce your chances of heart disease, slow down osteo-porosis, reduce your risk of cancer, fit into your favorite pair of jeans, not feel embarrassed at your next high school reunion or any other health and fitness benefit, you must first learn how.

Take the time to study how the body works. Just by read-ing this book you have already learned how your metabolism works and how to speed it permanently. However, this book is just the beginning. Continue your education and make sure you are gathering your information from credible sources. As I mentioned to Rob, don't go to the gym and copy others. You have no idea what their goals are and you are not experienced enough to know if what they are doing is correct. For me, it's comical. When I am traveling and need to go to a different health club or gym, I often see people copying others—and they are both performing the wrong exercises and doing them incorrectly! It is like the blind leading the blind!

If you are not 100 percent certain of how to do something, ask a qualified professional. Seek the advice of a certified per-sonal trainer and let him or her help you. And just like a med-ical doctor, if you feel that the advice the trainer provided you was not proper for what you want to do, get a second or third opinion. But whatever you do, don't just sit back and try to fig-ure it out on your own if you are not absolutely certain. You will either be doing the wrong things the wrong way and will not achieve the results you are working for or, worse yet, you will injure yourself and not be able to work out. You don't have to go it alone.

Read fitness books from credible and qualified sources. I know everyone has a "diet" on the market today, but filter through the garbage. You know by now that "dieting" doesn't work long-term and, worse yet, it ruins your metabolism permanently. Just because a pretty face or actor or actress is on the book cover, it doesn't mean the information is coming from a credible source. I know I am not telling you something you don't already know, but chances are the spokesperson or celebrity on the book cover had little if anything to do with the book. Believe it or not, book publishers want to make money and putting a recognizable and attractive person on the cover will help sell more books. That is why neither Don nor I put our faces on the cover of this book; we did not want to scare anyone off! A great place to buy informative books that you will not find at the local bookstore is Human Kinetics: www.humankinetics.com

Magazines are usually not as credible a source for unbiased information as books. The reason is because they have little time to gather information and like to change the content often so the magazine is different each issue. They also usually protect their advertisers by writing articles that support or at least do not deprecate their advertiser's products. Two magazines I highly recommend for mostly good and unbiased information are *The Journal of Strength and Condition Research*, available only through the National Strength and Condition Association, www.nsca-lift.org and *Personal Fitness Professional*. Learn the information personal trainers study at www.fit-pro.com.

Be very careful to filter any information from the Internet. Nearly every time I log on, I am greeted with a banner ad that promises me I can lose ten pounds in two weeks! Remember, diets don't work. Don't follow advice from some website that doesn't know you or your goals. Their claims are deceptive and their advice is misleading. I highly recommend that you ignore them altogether. Also, most of the fitness-related articles you see online are usually very vague and promote some type of diet or supplement. Others are somewhat better but usually written by fitness magazines that want you to become a subscriber.

For the best information on-line, I suggest the following: *The New England Journal of Medicine*, www.nejm.org; the Mayo Clinic, www.mayoclinic.com; and Pub Med, www.pubmed.com. These sites will give you the research and their findings. You are an intelligent person and don't need a pharmaceutical company or food manufacturer to tell you what to believe. See the research and read the conclusions for yourself. For new workout routines, I suggest www.testesterone.net and our site www.alessifit.com. I will again warn you to filter information you find on the Internet.

Spend the time to achieve peace of mind and grow closer to your fitness goals. Make an appointment with a personal trainer today. The information and knowledge will help you forever. You will never regret this decision; do it today.

Get Help!

SUMMARY

- Learn how your body and metabolism work by using a personal trainer.

- If you are not 100 percent certain of how to do something, ask a qualified professional.

- Filter through the garbage of fitness information in magazines, commercials, books, infomercials and online.

- You don't have to go it alone; get help!

PART II

A NEW LIFE

■

14

BEGIN YOUR TRANSFORMATION

I n the first three weeks of this system you will begin your transformation. The goal is to start to increase lean muscle tissue and get your metabolism moving. I don't want you to focus on your scale weight; rather, I want you to focus on your ability to burn fat and process food.

In this initial phase, you should learn to identify the real ingredients in foods and attempt to eat a supportive meal every three to three and a half hours. At first, if it is a challenge to eat every three hours, try to plan your meals in advance. When you get hungry, you'll eat whatever you can find if you haven't planned your meals. I suggest you plan meals for no less than one full day at a time. It's even better if you plan meals for the next two to three days in advance. Many of my private clients say this is the *single* biggest reason why they're able to eat well and reap the benefits of meal frequency and increased metabolism. I make it easy for my clients by having gourmet supportive meals available to them. A personal chef prepares these meals according to my criteria. The menu changes often and offers plain as well as exotic foods. They really have no excuse not to eat supportively!

Unfortunately, if you're expecting my brother Don or me to walk into your office with a hot plate of glazed turkey breast, sweet potatoes and lemon and herb green beans, you'd better not hold your breath! Seriously, though, if you have access to a refrigerator at work or if you can pack a small personal cooler, you have no excuse not to stick to the program. Please take the time to stock your refrigerator or cooler with supportive foods. Planning ahead really works and will accelerate your results.

Supplementation

A supplement is something that is used in addition to—not instead of—food. It's the "something extra." Many clients have asked me if a certain supplement is "worth it." I promise if you are not eating supportive nutrition every three to three and a half hours, increasing your lean muscle tissue and performing a moderate amount of cardiovascular training, no supplement is "worth it." Supplements will *not* work by themselves. The following is a synopsis of various supplements.

Essential Fatty Acids

If you're adhering to the Lose Fat Forever system, supplements will make the whole process more efficient. I strongly recommend consuming an essential fatty acid (EFA or omega-3 oils). Some of the best oils are flax or fish. Essential fatty acids help stabilize your blood sugar level, make your insulin receptors more efficient and satiate your body so you won't crave sugar. These oils are most effective in liquid, seed or ground forms rather than pills. My experience has shown that some people have trouble with the taste of the oil in liquid form. It's a "yuck" for them!

I suggest taking flax liquid with a chaser like a diet soda. It can also be blended into a protein shake, and some of my clients tell me they enjoy using it as a salad dressing.

Personally, I mix ground flax seeds in my oatmeal every morning and add a scoop of protein powder (more on that later). This provides a complete breakfast and is an effective way to consume flax. Follow the serving size on the container. Don't cook with EFA oils because the properties will be changed and you won't get their benefits.

EFAs are one of the best supplements to help you reach your goals of lowering your body fat and developing lean muscle tissue.

Post-Workout Protein Drinks

I recommend you consume a protein drink *immediately* after a weight training or cardiovascular training workout. On the days you perform both weight training and cardio, drink the protein shake at the end of the entire workout, not after each workout segment.

When you weight train, you create microscopic tears in muscle tissue. Remember, muscles are made of protein and protein is needed for muscle tissue to recuperate and repair itself. When muscle tissue is repaired, it becomes stronger and denser than it was initially, thus your body will develop muscle tissue. Consumption of post-workout protein helps this process.

A good protein supplement should be derived from a blend of whey, casein and egg protein. These types of protein promote the highest levels of protein assimilation (absorption into the body). If you're a strict vegetarian and don't wish to add protein sources from animal products, I suggest consuming soy protein powder. Though soy protein doesn't assimilate as well as a multi-blend of protein, it will help muscle tissue repair after weight training and is better than not consuming any protein post-workout.

Immediately after a weight training workout, your muscle cells are depleted of glycogen and best able to handle protein intake for their rebuilding. So as soon as you rack the weights, gulp a protein shake down! This will enhance development of your lean muscle tissue. Be sure to follow the serving size and directions on the package.

Many fitness professionals and scientists differ concerning the quantity of protein that can be absorbed at one time. I've read reports that suggest anywhere between twenty grams and 100 grams! Protein absorption will vary per individual based on size, amount of muscle tissue, age and activity level. While no one knows the exact protein absorbability, I personally suggest you consume a minimum of twenty-five grams in your post-workout shake. Contact a nutritionist if you have additional questions about protein consumption. Check out our website, www.AlessiFit.com, for a list of recommended meal replacement and protein shakes.

L-Glutamine

Your muscle is composed of twenty-two amino acids, one of which is L-Glutamine. Remember, the only way to increase your metabolism permanently is to increase your lean muscle tissue. When muscle tissue is broken down through resistance training, it needs to repair, regenerate and grow stronger. L-Glutamine is important in its ability to repair and recuperate muscle tissue. L-Glutamine is also vital in allowing your immune system to operate effectively and helps prevent illnesses.

L-Glutamine is available naturally through most meat and poultry protein sources. However, L-Glutamine is best if taken in powder form following your workout. As with the post workout protein drink, the body will absorb L-Glutamine into the muscles and cells immediately after they have been broken down and are in a catabolic state. It is impractical and inefficient to attempt to eat meat after you finish your weight training, so add L-Glutamine powder to your post workout protein drink. I have personally experienced the benefits of L-Glutamine powder within two workouts. You will feel stronger and encounter less muscular fatigue.

Meal Replacement Shakes

If you travel often and *don't* have access to a refrigerator or a cooler of food from home, I suggest you carry a meal replacement shake, which should consist of a balance of proteins, carbohydrates and some essential fats. Your muscles and your metabolism need this nourishment for development. The difference between a meal replacement shake and a protein shake is that a meal replacement shake is a "meal replacement." A protein shake does not contain carbohydrates or fats and is most effective immediately following a workout. A meal replacement shake can be consumed anytime in place of a meal.

I'm not suggesting if you don't travel that you cannot have or shouldn't have a meal replacement shake. You can absolutely have a meal replacement shake at home or the office. They can be an acceptable substitute for real food, especially if you're not going to eat otherwise. However, if you have the choice, *always* opt for real food. Also, make sure your meal replacement shake doesn't contain saturated fats and hydrogenated oils and has very few (less than three) grams of simple sugars per serving.

Protein Bars

Marketers are having a field day selling protein bars. They're found in most health food stores, grocery stores, department stores and even gas stations! Protein bars should be eaten only when you *do not* have access to real food. They're only useful in keeping your metabolism moving when you wouldn't eat otherwise. I predict that they will become less popular in the coming years when consumers discover the actual contents of the bars.

The nutritional content of protein bars is typically *not* what the manufacturer claims on the label. First, protein has a limited shelf life. If a label on a bar claims that it contains forty grams of protein, this means that it had forty grams of protein at the time it was manufactured. Often, it has much less protein by the time you eat it several months later.

Secondly, bar manufacturers often use a product called glycerin or glycerol as a sweetener. Glycerol is a sugar; however, it is an alcohol sugar. The Food and Drug Administration (FDA) doesn't require alcohol byproducts to be listed on food labels. So, manufacturers can claim their bar contains "zero carbohydrates," even when it's sweetened with glycerol or other simple sugars such as aorbitol, xylitol and mannitol. These sugars will react in your body the same way as sucrose or fructose. Thus you believe you're eating a supportive protein source when in actuality, you're eating a dry candy bar! Remember, you can always locate these sugars on the ingredients list.

Dawn Jackson, RD, spokeswomen for the American Dietetic Association states, "Some of the (protein) bars have as much sugar and as much saturated fat as a candy bar. So use them in moderation." In October 2001, ConsumerLab.com conducted an independent study of protein bars. Their laboratory tests revealed that eighteen of the thirty bars they tested did not meet the claims of ingredient levels printed on the label. Their findings went on to expose that half of the tested bars exceeded the carbohydrate grams stated on the label. In fact, one bar that promoted itself as a low carbohydrate bar claimed it had just two grams of carbohydrates, but the test revealed that it contained twenty-two grams! That is a difference of twenty grams or five teaspoons of sugar!

Try to eliminate protein or energy bars. You won't get the nourishment your muscle tissue needs for development and the hidden sugar will sabotage your goals. A meal replacement shake is a better alternative than a protein bar for supportive nutrition. Always, real food is the best choice.

The importance of water

I recommend you drink a minimum of half your body weight in ounces of water. For example, if you weigh 160 pounds, drink eighty ounces of water a day. Get a sixteen-ounce water bottle, fill it up and drink it five times a day. Remember, if you want to speed up your metabolism, it's very important to develop lean muscle tissue. Since muscle tissue is roughly composed of eighty percent water, it behooves you to increase your water intake. The more water your muscles can hold, the more muscle you will have.

Any type of cell in your body needs only two elements to be healthy and grow: oxygen and water. If you nourish your cells properly, they will become healthier and stronger. In your muscle tissue, adequate water intake facilitates recuperation and development more efficiently and to a greater extent than is possible without adequate water intake.

Water also dilutes toxins in your body. If you recall from high school biology class, respiration occurs within your cells and results in the production of carbon dioxide. Water is fundamental in transporting carbon dioxide and other toxins away from the cells, thus assisting your blood in cell purification. Further, water helps muscle hydration, which in turn enhances muscle endurance.

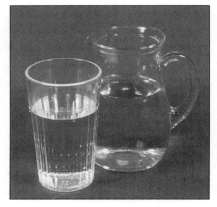

Drink a minimum of half your body weight in ounces of water daily.

A good rule to remember is that the more muscle tissue you have and the larger you are, the more water you should drink. Also, it's necessary to consume a generous amount of water after exercise to rehydrate your body. Your body will naturally lose water during a workout.

It's important not to drink too much water during your workout. Excess water will swish around in your stomach and make you feel sick, and can potentially lead to abdominal cramping. I've witnessed hundreds of individuals consume too much water during workouts, only to feel sluggish and sick. As I tell my clients, drink water sparingly during the workout and then *drink until you float* after the workout.

Please note: water intake means pure water. Water contained in coffee, tea and soda or sugar-based drinks is *not* pure water! Most of these beverages will do more to dehydrate you than to adequately hydrate your body. I'm not saying that you cannot drink coffee or tea, just realize they don't count toward your desired water intake.

One last thought on water: unless you are an athlete or are competing in endurance events, please don't drink Gatorade or other sports drinks. I know the commercials for these products make you think their product is better than water because it replaces vitamins and minerals you excrete when working out. Unless you are an athlete, you probably won't lose that many vitamins and minerals during your workout. These drinks contain a very high concentration of simple sugars, which can turn to fat in your body. Water is a much better alternative to achieving your goal of decreasing body fat.

Sleep

When resistance training is performed, muscle is broken down and microscopic tears occur in the tissue. In order for the tissue to develop stronger and increase tone and endurance, the body needs to repair. Repair occurs through nutrition, hydration and rest. I have already covered the first two, so let's focus on rest. While many strategies exist for active rest, such as massage, hydrotherapy, thermo treatments and meditation, arguably the most effective method of recovery, sleep, is often neglected.

There are five distinct states of sleep: stages one, two, three, four, and REM (rapid eye movement). The most important for recovery and rest are stages three and four, which are often grouped together and referred to as slow-wave sleep, and REM. Two physiological events occur during slow-wave sleep that aid recovery. First, metabolic activity is lowest. The body utilizes the least amount of energy in this phase. For recovery purposes, this is beneficial. The body will stop all but the most essential functions so that repair and development can be maximized.

Secondly, the endocrine system increases the secretion of growth hormone from the pituitary gland. This aids in the rebuilding of all tissues, especially muscle tissue. Moore and LeVert, in their book *The Complete Idiot's Guide to Getting a Good Night's Sleep*, reveal the benefits of growth hormone release on tissue repair through a demonstration in skin tissue, which they claim multiplies at "twice its normal rate during slow-wave sleep."

A sleep deficit or deprivation will impair your body's ability to develop lean muscle tissue. This will reduce your muscle tone, strength and metabolism. Also, sleep deficit individuals show difficulty containing anger and commonly display increased levels of depression, stress, anxiety, worry and frustration.

The exact amount of sleep required for every individual varies. The frequent recommendation that you need to sleep at least eight hours per night is too simplistic and inaccurate. For example, Dan Jansen, the 1994 men's Olympic gold medallist in speed skating, slept an average of ten hours per night. Bonnie Blair, the women's gold medallist in speed skating, slept little more than six hours per night during the same Olympics.

One method to help determine your required amount of sleep is to be aware of and follow your circadian rhythms. Circadian rhythms are your internal clock that determines when you naturally feel alert or sleepy. For example, I wake up early and always feel strong throughout the morning and early part of the day. Even on my day off, I have a hard time staying in bed after 5:30 am. However, I usually begin to feel sleepy around 9 p.m and get to bed at 10 p.m. Most importantly, circadian rhythms need consistency to perform efficiently. You must wakeup and go to sleep within one hour of your usual time each day.

Some shift workers have a very erratic schedule. They rotate their work shifts where they alternate work between days and nights, never developing a consistent sleep pattern. Consequently, shift workers report more difficulty sleeping than any other subset group in the nation. According to research performed at the Institute for Circadian Physiology in Boston, nearly seventy percent of shift workers report trouble sleeping. Dr. Martin Moore-Ede, sleep specialist at the University of Harvard Medical School and author of *The Twenty-Four Hour Society*, states that "changing one's schedule for more than two days or sleeping more than one hour longer on the weekends disrupts the biological clock." Other experts believe that people feel tired and lethargic on Mondays because they have changed their biological clock drastically over the weekend.

By altering your wake-up and bedtime significantly on the weekend, when Monday morning comes around, your body will be seeking more sleep. Statistically, more heart attacks and strokes occur on Monday than all the other days of the week combined. Many experts believe this is a direct effect of altering sleep behavior on the weekends. Unneeded stress and pressure is placed on your system.

I strongly encourage you to keep the same sleep schedule on the weekends. I know how tempting it is to sleep in. However, if you "suck it up and fall out of bed," you will feel better throughout the day and sleep better at night. You will also not loathe Monday morning like you do now. You will feel refreshed and strong. You will also strengthen you immune system and have fewer sleeping problems. Most importantly, you will repair you lean muscle tissue, burn more calories, increase your metabolism and look and feel better. Get to sleep!

Protein Day

After you have conditioned your body to exercising and eating supportive nutrition for the first three weeks, I introduce a "protein day" into the system. The protein day is designed to accelerate the reduction of your body fat. I still want you to continue to eat every three to three and a half hours; however, you should *not* consume a slow-releasing carbohydrate on protein days. Instead, I want you to eat a larger serving (one and a half times the size of your fist) of protein and green vegetables so your body doesn't undergo calorie deprivation.

On non-weight training days, your body will be forced to use fat for energy if the amount of sugar (both simple and complex) in your body is reduced. Don't eliminate slow-releasing complex carbohydrates on weight training days because your body will need them for sustained energy levels. Although vegetables contain complex carbohydrates, the high amount of fiber contained in vegetables is helpful in aiding body fat reduction and promotes satiation or "fullness."

Sometimes clients ask me about the amount of protein grams that should be consumed in a day. There's no easy way to answer this question. Overall, macronutrient consumption (protein, carbs or fats) depends upon fitness goals, body size, age and other health considerations. However, I want to remind you that lean protein is not calorically dense. For example, 100 grams of a lean protein source is equivalent to 400 calories. Most adults should be able to easily consume 400 calories of protein a day. If you want to simplify your life, forget all macronutrient grams and use your fist as a guide as I mentioned in Chapter 4. This way you will be eating a small amount of lean protein five times a day.

Fiber

Fiber is classified as either soluble or insoluble. Both types are important and necessary to a balanced and supportive nutrition plan.

Soluble fiber helps reduce cholesterol. Examples of soluble fiber are oats, oat bran, oatmeal, beans, peas and barley. Oats have a greater proportion of soluble fiber than any other grain.

Insoluble fiber is important in promoting normal bowel functions and digestion. Insoluble fiber includes whole-wheat breads, wheat cereals, wheat bran, rye and most other whole grains.

The American Heart Association (AHA) suggests eating a variety of foods to obtain fiber. The AHA in its medical article, "Fiber, Lipids, and Coronary Heart Disease," states, "Total dietary intake should be 25–30 grams a day (of fiber)." Further, the AHA suggests that it is desirable to "intake of both types of fiber in a ratio of one part soluble to three parts insoluble fiber."

Recent AHA findings indicate that fiber also reduces the risk of obesity: "It has been hypothesized that high-fiber foods may favorably impact satiety and slow gastric emptying, thereby sustaining a feeling of fullness that prohibits overeating. Intake of high-fiber foods may also improve glycemic control in diabetic individuals and reduce risk of insulin resistance."

Other positive benefits of fiber include reducing low density lipoproteins (LDL, "bad" cholesterol) and blood pressure. Lastly, the AHA warns that, "Many commercial oat bran and wheat bran products (muffins, chips, waffles) actually contain very little bran." It's important to stay with foods like oatmeal (whole grain) and whole wheat bread.

In the Lose Fat Forever system, you will eat foods high in both soluble and insoluble fiber. This will help you attain all of the above benefits. In addition to eating whole foods containing fiber, I also suggest you take an insoluble fiber supplement once a day. I recommend guar gum in either pill or powder form. Follow the directions on the label and consult with your physician if you have any questions. Another product new on the market is Fiber-Psyll, manufactured by MD Labs. It contains guar gum, potato fiber and protein as well as other fibers into one package. Adequate fiber intake helps digestion, lowers cholesterol, blood pressure and your body fat.

Multi-Vitamins

Vitamins are the catalysts that allow metabolic processes to occur. Research has shown that certain vitamins act as anti-oxidants, which help neutralize and eliminate toxins and free radicals in your body. Most Americans can benefit by taking a quality multi-vitamin daily because they do not consume enough vitamins in their food. In fact, the food consumed by most Americans is vitamin-deficient and nutritionally pitiful. However, now that you are eating a lean protein source, a slow-releasing carbohydrate and a green vegetable frequently and using an essential fatty acid like flax oil once a day, you will not be vitamin-deficient. My suggestion is that you take a multi-vitamin once a day as an insurance policy to complement the supportive eating habits I have taught you.

Day's End

I'm often asked, "What time should I stop eating for the day?" Again, there is no easy answer. You must first consider your goals. If you want to lose body fat, I share the opinion of many other fitness professionals when I recommend you stop eating within three hours of bedtime. Your body doesn't need or use many calories while you are sleeping. So if you provide fuel for your body and perform no activity to utilize the fuel, your body will store it as fat.

If your goal is to increase muscle mass and size and you don't have a major concern with body fat reduction, it's advisable to eat a protein source before bedtime. This is because your body will break down protein and muscle tissue while you sleep. In order to prevent or slow down this protein catabolization, you should consume some type of lean protein source, like cottage cheese, before bedtime. Remember, do this only if you are *not concerned* about losing body fat.

15

QUESTIONS AND ANSWERS

Q: What if I don't have enough time to exercise?

A: I've heard this one for years. Well guess what—neither Don nor I have the time, either! I have a clientele that includes physicians, attorneys, financial planners, professors, CEOs and the mayor, and none of these people have the time to exercise. In fact, I've never had the privilege of hearing a client say to me, "Derek, I would really love to get into shape and I have all the time in the world. Could you train me and give me something to do to help me occupy my days?"

Probably, no one has the time to exercise and eat supportive meals frequently. However, human beings will make the time for things that they believe are important. If you're unwilling to make time for your health and fitness, they are clearly not your highest priority.

As I mentioned in earlier, I personally train many financially wealthy clients who have neglected their health to build their wealth and then attempt to use their wealth to buy back their health. Often they are unsuccessful at reversing the effects of obesity, diabetes, heart disease, osteoporosis and chronic fatigue. Every one of these clients tells me the same thing: "I wish I would have taken better care of my health and fitness sooner." This is a sad situation in which many individuals find themselves. Remember, no one ever said at the end of his or her life, "I wish I had spent more time at the office!"

Q: Am I too old?

A: No!—unless you're no longer moving, breathing or processing food. Don and I have worked with clients well into their late eighties! If they can do it, you can do it, too. As mentioned earlier, I advise you to check with your physician or health care professional before starting an exercise program, especially if you believe your health may be in question.

I do believe that your health and fitness goals should be consistent with your age. For example, I wouldn't begin a program designed to promote dramatic body fat reduction with someone who is eighty years old. However, I believe someone that age in good health can improve their lean muscle mass, strength and endurance. This will help them feel and move better, as well as increasing bone density. It's never too late to start.

Q: I've never stuck with an exercise program before. Am I doomed to fail?

A: You're only doomed if you believe that you are. Your mental attitude toward health and fitness is extremely important. If you believe you can follow this system, you will. If you believe you cannot follow this system or any other, you won't. Success or failure depends upon you.

I believe this system is more complete than most others. As I stated in the introduction, other "diets" you may have tried use a "trick" that couldn't possibly work for the long run. So, you didn't fail; the "diet" or "quick fix" plan failed you. Try the Lose Fat Forever system, complete all the workouts and nutritional recommendations, and I promise you great success in accomplishing your goals.

Q: I don't like to exercise. What else can I do?

A: I wish I could wave a magic wand and you could get all the benefits of exercise without ever having to break a sweat. In fact, marketers of many diet pills, electro-stimulation machines, ab rollers and infomercial gadgets know Americans want the easy way out and *prey* on it. They claim their product gives you all the benefits of exercise and proper nutrition without you ever having to lift a finger or change your behavior. These claims are misleading, deceptive and, in many cases, outright bogus. The goal of these phony products and gadgets is to make money. I think by now you know that improving your health and fitness by use of these products is impossible. The only thing that will be thinner after you purchase these products will be your wallet!

I know many of my clients don't like to exercise, but they do it and are committed to it because it helps them feel better and look better. They also value their health and want to prevent the occurrence of lifestyle-related diseases. I'm not asking you to quit your job and become a personal trainer, and I realize for some of you, exercise is not the pinnacle of your day. However, with a focused system and appropriate goals, I believe you may appreciate the value of exercise and do it even if it isn't your favorite thing. Your workouts will be challenging and changing constantly. The time you spend exercising will be effective and move you closer to your goals in an efficient manner.

Q: Am I too fat?

A: No! Don and I have helped dozens people to lose more than 100 pounds of fat and dramatically transform their life. We've seen hundreds of people lose more than fifty pounds of fat, increase their lean muscle mass and reduce their waistlines in half. You're never too fat to undertake a program to improve. However, I want you to realize the more fat you have, the longer it will take to accomplish your goals. But, as long as you are alive, there's still time to improve your health and fitness. I usually set a goal with my clients to reduce their body fat by two to four percent a month. This can be reasonably accomplished by following the Lose Fat Forever system.

Q: I've tried other programs before and they didn't work. How is this one different?

A: As I said before, you didn't fail, miracle "diets" and fat loss products you may have tried failed *you*. By reading this far, you've learned how your body works. You now know that any system that doesn't contain steps for developing lean muscle tissue, supportive nutrition, and moderate cardiovascular training is incomplete and doomed to fail. My system includes all of these components necessary for success. This is the only complete system that ever took the time to educate you on how your body works.

Q: Will weight lifting make me look too bulky?

A: No. I know many women, and some men, are worried about becoming big and bulky. If you don't want to look big and bulky you need to lose body fat and develop your lean muscle tissue. Muscle tissue is lean and takes up almost four times less space than fat! A pound of fat takes up as much room as your clenched fist, whereas a pound of lean muscle tissue takes up as much room as a silver dollar. Unless you are into taking male hormones and steroids and spending four hours a day in the gym, there is *absolutely no way* you'll ever look like a body builder. Weight training and body fat reduction will make you appear lean and healthy.

Q: Why should I exercise if I can just take a pill that will increase my metabolism?

A: You need to be aware there is no such thing as a "magic pill" that will increase your metabolism. Remember, your metabolism is the rate at which your body processes and utilizes fuel. Only the development of lean muscle tissue, supportive nutrition and moderate cardiovascular training will increase the rate at which your body processes fuel. You may buy pills that claim they are metabolism enhancers, however, you will *only* increase your heart rate. These pills are *dangerous* and won't work for the long run, even if you lose water weight initially.

The reason you could initially lose weight with these pills is because your heart is a pump. If you increase the speed at which your heart pumps, it will extract more water out of your system, but this isn't the excess water that your body stores in your bladder. It is water located in your muscles, internal organs and cells.

You now know that your muscle tissue is composed of nearly eighty percent water, so if you decrease the water content in your muscle tissue, you'll have less muscle tissue. Less muscle tissue will lead to a slower metabolism. Consequently, taking pills you believe will increase your metabolism will actually have the opposite effect in the long run!

"Metabolism increasing" pills can also potentially be dangerous. They often have side effects that include dizziness, jitteriness, headaches and inability to concentrate. Increased pressure on your heart may also result from the ability of these pills to elevate blood pressure and speed heart rate. Since many of these pills contain "the stack," a mixture of caffeine, ephedrine and aspirin, they can be addictive.

You may have heard that a popular "metabolism increasing" pill, Metabolife, has come under criminal investigation recently. The Justice Department has revealed that more than

13,000 health complaints have come against this product. A reported eighty of these claims involve serious disease or death, and 100 to 200 others deal with people being hospitalized. Metabolife is the biggest offender, but clearly not the only one on the market.

Any product or pill that promises to burn fat or increase your metabolism is bogus, deceptive and misleading. And worse than that, it is dangerous. These products and pills will soon be illegal and taken off the market but, unfortunately, not soon enough.

Caffeine and ephedrine are stimulants; they will artificially increase your heart rate. Together they act as a small dosage of speed. Aspirin will thin your blood and increase the rate at which the stimulants enter your body. Since your goal is to increase your *health* and fitness. Avoid these products.

Q: Do fat blockers work to help reduce body fat and weight?

A: No! "Fat blockers" have not been proven to work in reducing body fat. The only thing they block is necessary, essential dietary fat from properly nourishing your body. Remember, consumption of dietary fat is not the only way a person gains weight. As you've learned through reading my system, you could become very fat even if you don't consume *any* dietary fat. If you consume excess sugar or even excess protein, your body will convert what you don't use to body fat.

Dietary fat and body fat aren't the same. Some types of unsaturated dietary fat are an essential macronutrient that you must consume to be healthy and for body processes to function normally. Body fat is the accumulation of excess adipose tissue, produced by your body's inability to utilize your ingestion of food.

If you use a *legitimate* "fat blocker" (obtained with a prescription, not through an infomercial!), they don't work either.

You will most likely become deficient in essential fatty acids (dietary fat) with these products. When this happens, your body will break down muscle tissue to provide itself with essential fats and you will lose lean muscle tissue. This reduction of lean muscle tissue will slow down your metabolism and increase your body fat in the long run.

Further, many prescription fat blockers are associated with undesirable side effects, for example, changes in bowel habits, gas with discharge, an urgent need to go to the bathroom, oily or fatty stools, an oily discharge, increased number of bowel movements and an inability to control bowel movements. Not what I would call a fun evening! Fat blockers are bogus and don't work. Avoid them and save your doctor the embarrassment.

Q: What would happen if I just stop eating to lose weight?

A: You'll become fatter! If you stop eating, you'll lose water and lean muscle tissue. Muscle tissue is the only place in your body that burns fat and calories, so if you lose muscle, you'll slow down your body's ability to burn fat and calories. The initial decrease in your scale weight will soon be replaced by the addition of body fat and your metabolism will slow down. You'll condition yourself to be fatter, and you'll also be hungry and more apt to binge eat. Don't stop eating!

Q: I'm not sure I have the willpower to get in shape. How can I stick to this system?

A: You must *decide* to stick to this system. It's not a matter of will power; it's a matter of commitment. You must commit yourself to:

- Improving your health and fitness.
- Following and completing the system.
- Becoming the best you have ever been.

If you can't dedicate yourself to these goals, there isn't a program in existence that will help you.

If you are willing to dedicate yourself to and follow the Lose Fat Forever system, I promise you'll achieve better health and fitness than you ever imagined possible. A healthy and fit attitude often creates internal momentum that will enable you to achieve your health and fitness goals.

Q: Am I just predestined to be fat?

A: No! I don't doubt genetic factors may be involved at some level in the development of muscle or fatty tissue. Children who grow up with parents who are obese have a tendency to become obese themselves. Often, the obesity link between parents and children has to do more with poor parental role modeling and behavior than DNA. However, the genetic tendency to be overweight can be modified if you commit yourself to developing lean muscle tissue, eating supportive meals and performing cardiovascular training in moderation.

I tell my clients, "It isn't your genes that are making you out of shape and unhealthy; it's your behavior." After I adjust the eating and exercise behavior of my clients, they no longer regard their genes as an obstacle or an excuse. When you practice lifestyle modification by following my system, you'll be surprised at how little genetic differences actually matter.

Q: I don't want to compromise the quality of my life by worrying about not eating and drinking items that I enjoy. Despite this, I still want to get into better health and fitness. Is it possible?

A: Yes! When you engage in the Lose Fat Forever system, you'll find you don't have to compromise the things you enjoy in your life. You've decided to take charge and live your life and this will create enjoyment. When you dedicate yourself to this system, you won't feel deprived; you'll feel proud of yourself for making the changes to improve your health and fitness.

You're an interesting and exciting person. You're so much more than junk food and alcohol. Don't believe that by limiting your consumption of certain foods and beverages, life won't be worth living. Remember, you can have whatever you desire in moderation on your "cheat day." You'll feel and move better. You'll be able to do things that were physically impossible before. And you'll look better than you have in years. Your quality of life will improve; it will not be compromised!

Q: I've read other books that tell me to "just love the real me" and not worry about my shape. How do you feel about that?

A: I believe that self-respect and self-confidence are extremely important. However, I don't think the premise of those books is to promote complacency and neglect your health and fitness. I believe they're trying to inform you that you don't have to look like a supermodel to feel worthy.

The Lose Fat Forever system is based upon the theory that you can gain self-respect by improving your health and fitness while practicing an enjoyable lifestyle. Most individuals aren't aiming to be supermodels or professional athletes. This system is for regular people like you and me who have limited time each day to spend on health and fitness. It allows for achieving maximum health and fitness in an efficient manner.

Q: Why do I have to follow this system for eighteen weeks when I saw an advertisement that read "Lose thirty pounds in thirty days"? Is there a quicker way?

A: No! Remember, there are no short cuts to permanently lowering your body fat and fat weight. The advertisement you see on telephone poles or in commercials are usually promoting some "magic pill" that is supposed to increase your metabolism. As I said before, metabolism enhancers don't exist. Only weight training, supportive nutrition and moderate cardiovascular training will increase your metabolism. These magic pills will do no more than artificially raise your heart rate. In fact, ask yourself this question: "If these products worked so well, why wouldn't everyone who used them be in great shape?

The speed of your results depends on your goals and your fitness when you start the system. For example, if your goal is to lower your body fat two percent, you could probably accomplish this goal in one month. If you've never exercised before and you want to lose twenty percent body fat, seventy-five pounds of scale weight and drop six dress or suit sizes, You probably need to give yourself a reasonable timetable of at least twelve to fifteen months.

Q. Do electrical muscle stimulation machines work to cut fat on my abs?

A. No. Electrical muscle stimulation (EMS) has been used by physical therapists for years as a method to rehabilitate neuro-muscular connections after injury or surgery. Recently, advertisers have been bombarding commercials, infomercials, magazine, newspapers and other media with claims that EMS decreases body fat, increases strength, shapes and tones your muscles and helps you chisel the body of your dreams!

Scientists at the University of Wisconsin, Department of Exercise and Sports Science and Department of Physical Therapy, studied the effects of EMS machines per manufacturers claims. The researchers had subjects use the machine three times per week for eight weeks, following the manufacturers recommendations. Testing protocols measured changes in body fat, fat weight, lean body mass, girth measurements and strength. At the end of the study, the researchers found, "The EMS had no significant effects on any of the measured parameters. Thus, claims relative to the effectiveness of the EMS for the apparent healthy individual are not supported by the findings of this study." So in other words, the machine did nothing to reduce fat or increase muscle. In fact, the participants in the study actually gained body fat and fat weight while using the machine! If you have already purchased one of these devices, I'm sorry, but it will not help you lose body fat, inches, fat weight or increase strength.

Q. What percentage does my body fat have to be in order to see my abs?
A. For men, eight to ten percent and for women ten to twelve percent. The only way to visually see definition in your abs or in any muscle group is to have low body fat. Remember, no matter what commercials say, it is impossible to spot reduce any area of the body. So do not train your abs with a different agenda than the rest of your body.

Q: Does liposuction work? If so, why can't I have it done instead of following this system?

A: Liposuction is a painful short-term surgical solution to a long-term behavioral problem. If you need a physician to suction fat out of your body with a vacuum, your health and fitness level will not be improved. You will have done nothing to improve your muscle tone, metabolism, strength, health, endurance, cardiovascular stamina and lifestyle behavior. In fact, most reputable plastic surgeons won't even perform this procedure on the casual individual looking to lose some fat.

Furthermore, you may look disproportionate. You can't have body fat removed from every site on your body simultaneously. You can have your tummy and hips done, but you may still have fat on your face, neck and back. Also, fat is a cell. Like all cells in your body, fat will divide and multiply.

If you give blood, you're not permanently short one pint of blood; your body will produce more blood cells. If you cut your hand, your body will produce more skin cells. If you have a tummy tuck and don't change the habits and lifestyle that led you to need the procedure, your body will produce more fat cells as well!

I recently read an advertisement for a group of plastic surgeons who were performing a free seminar for individuals interested in liposuction and "body contouring." The seminar discussed the process involved with the surgery. Reservations were required and refreshments of *wine, cheese and desserts* were served!

You need to treat the problem, not the short-term symptom. The Lose Fat Forever system will teach you how to take control of your health and fitness for good. With this system, you'll learn how to lower your body fat permanently without having to go under the knife. And you'll improve so much more than just your appearance.

Q: Do women need a workout and nutritional program that is different from a man's?

A: Yes! However, the principles are the same. Both men and women need to learn to take control of their metabolism. Both need to develop lean muscle tissue, eat supportive meals frequently and perform a moderate amount of cardiovascular training.

In the ten years that I've been a personal fitness professional, I've learned women can't lift as much weight as men. (It really didn't take me that long to realize it!) Also, a woman should consume fewer calories than a man because she has a smaller amount of lean muscle tissue. However, the principles in the Lose Fat Forever system apply equally to both men and women.

Q: How can I consult with you or Don for health and fitness advice?

A: Both Don and I work in our private training facilities in the Buffalo New York area. You can call our office, e-mail or write.

We conduct telephone as well as in-office consultations, and we also specialize in corporate seminars.

Derek Alessi
7662 Transit Road
Williamsville NY 14221
(716) 635-0758
ThePromise@alessifit.com

Don Alessi
300 Delaware Avenue
Buffalo NY 14202
(716) 853-4930
D_Strength@hotmail.com

16

WORDS OF ENCOURAGEMENT

've enjoyed furthering your education about health, fitness and how your body works. I trust you found this book informative and motivational. As I mentioned at the beginning of this book, it doesn't matter if you are male or female. It doesn't matter if you are eighteen or eighty years old. It doesn't matter if you have ever been in shape before or ever stuck with an organized exercise plan for more than the two weeks after a New Year's resolution. You *have* the power to transform your health and fitness. As a result, you'll benefit from increased energy and productivity. You'll also be able to wear clothes that reveal your new shape. Most importantly, remember you have the power to increase your enjoyment of life!

You've learned how to take control of your nutritional habits and not be deceived by misleading food marketers, and gained understanding of the fraud behind fitness claims and radical diets. I have confidence you now have the basic tools you need to empower yourself and take control of your body. I'm also confident you've increased your self-confidence, self-respect and sense of personal empowerment through adhering to my 100 percent effective system.

If this is the first time you've been exposed to this information, I encourage you to read it again or call for a personal fitness consultation. Don and I look forward to helping anyone who is serious about improving his or her health and fitness. Are you ready to begin?

As I said earlier, *do not* begin this program unless you are absolutely committed to:

- Improving your health and fitness.
- Following and completing the system.
- Becoming the best you have ever been.

Once you've done this, you'll attain every fitness goal you set out to accomplish. You'll look and feel the way you desire. You will have transformed your health and fitness!

On the following pages I have outlined my plan for the next 126 days. Follow these steps as if you were following a treasure map that leads you to gold.

You'll be beginning a new exercise program. Included are pictures and descriptions of exercises, as well as the workouts themselves. Remember, always use weight that you can handle. It's better to start light and increase weight as needed, than to use weights you can't handle and do it wrong. Our website, www.AlessiFit.com, visually demonstrates with streaming video how to perform all the exercises properly. If you have any questions about the workouts or exercises, please contact a personal fitness professional.

I'm going to ask you to do some additional cardiovascular training on some of your non-weight training days. On these days, it's important to do your cardio at a moderate pace. I define a moderate pace as being a level six or seven out of ten, with ten being the most difficult. Please don't go too fast or exceed the time I recommend. Remember, I don't want you to mentally burn out or break down muscle tissue.

I'm also going to ask you to rate your performance each day on a scale from one to ten, with one being the least effort you could possibly imagine and ten being your maximal effort. I don't expect you to be perfect every day; I know you're human. However, I want you to be as conscientious as possible. You need an honest evaluation of your effort for your own feedback. Your results will always parallel your effort. If you perform at a high rate for the day and the week, it will show in the results.

It's very important to rate yourself honestly. It won't benefit you if you give yourself a higher score than you deserve. So rate yourself honestly and accurately. Your good effort will shine through!

I can only educate you so much—now it's time for you to execute. Good luck and stay committed to the plan. Your results depend upon it!

LOSE FAT FOREVER SUMMARY

- If you want to reduce your body fat for the rest of your life, never diet again.

- When you "diet" you condition your body to burn less fat and fewer calories.

- SYNERGY is the only way to permanently increase your metabolism.

- SYNERGY involves 1) developing lean muscle tissue 2) increasing the frequency of eating supportive meals and 3) performing a moderate amount of cardiovascular exercise.

- When you develop lean muscle tissue, you produce heat, which has a metabolic effect of burning fat and calories

- The more lean muscle tissue you have, the faster your metabolism will work.

- Lean muscle tissue takes up four times less space than fatty tissue.

- Eat a supportive meal every three to three and a half hours.

- The more frequently you eat, the more conditioned and efficient your body will become to burning food.

- A supportive meal contains a lean protein, a slow-releasing carbohydrate, and a vegetable (preferably green).

- Proteins are essential and provide twice as much thermal effect as carbohydrates or fats.

- Protein is necessary for the development of lean muscle tissue and ridding the body of fat.

- Incorporate one "cheat day" into your supportive eating habits.

- On your cheat day, eat whatever you want, in moderation.

- The body requires essential fatty acids (EFAs) such as flax and fish oils, not saturated fats and hydrogenated oils.

- One gram of fat contains nine calories!

- Sugar causes an insulin response that ultimately leads to fat gain.

- Always check the ingredients list of foods so that you are less likely to be deceived by slick marketers.

- Consume no more than two servings of alcohol per week.

- Fruit is a simple sugar, so limit your consumption.

- Look at product labels to see if manufacturers are "sneaking" fats and sugars into the ingredients lists.

- Consuming too much sugar or fat will increase your body fat and jeopardize your health and fitness goals.

- Performing too much cardiovascular training may break down your muscle tissue. This will slow down your metabolism and make you fatter.

- Spend less time doing cardiovascular training and more time engaging in weight training.

- Contact a personal fitness professional if you have questions regarding weight training or cardiovascular training workouts.

- If you don't change your workout often, you will plateau.

- Following the Lose Fat Forever system will constantly challenge your muscles to adapt to different stimuli by employing workout variation.

- Don't fool yourself into thinking you'll begin to work out tomorrow, next month or after the holidays. Do it now!

- Every day you procrastinate is another day further from your goals, dreams and better health.

- There is no such thing as the perfect time!

There is nothing training cannot do.
Nothing is above its reach.
It can turn bad morals to good;
it can destroy bad principles
and recreate good ones;
it can lift men to angelship.

—MARK TWAIN

PART III

TIME TO EAT

■

17

SAMPLE MEAL PLANS AND GROCERY LIST

T he following chart shows a sample day of supportive nutrition. If you have any questions regarding these meals or types of foods, consult with a nutritionist or dietician in your area.

You will notice meals are spaced three hours apart. It is essential you eat every three to three and a half hours to speed up your metabolism. Substitute any protein, slow-releasing carbohydrate and vegetable with any item listed on the second chart of supportive foods.

Sample Day of Supportive Nutrition

7 a.m.	Breakfast	Egg white omelet with wheat toast, flax seeds, guar gum fiber.
10 a.m.	Snack	Cottage cheese (1%) and whole wheat crackers
1 p.m.	Lunch	Grilled chicken over a bed of leafy lettuce, veggies and a sweet potato
4 p.m.	Snack	Meal replacement shake
7 p.m.	Dinner	Chicken/steak/fish with brown rice and veggies

Next, here is a list of some of the most common supportive foods:

Supportive Foods

Lean proteins	Slow-releasing carbohydrates	Vegetables
Egg whites	Wheat bread	Broccoli
Egg Beaters	Wheat pasta	Spinach
Chicken breast	Sweet potatoes/yams	Green beans
Turkey breast	Oatmeal	Asparagus
Steak	Brown rice	Mushrooms
Fish	Wild rice	Cauliflower
Shellfish	Whole grain couscous	Leafy lettuce
Cottage cheese (1%)		Peppers
Ostrich		
Pork		
Veal		
Buffalo (not the city)		
Tuna		
Protein powders		
Tofu		

Note: foods can be substituted

Quick and easy meal suggestions

Below I have included samples of my own supportive nutrition meals that can be used as a guide. I know you don't have a lot of time to plan your nutrition, so I'm not going to give you elaborate recipes that call for dozens of ingredients and several measuring cups. These are supportive meal combinations that can be prepared easily.

Derek's favorites

I usually wake up at 4 a.m. (I have a dedicated and early-rising clientele) and make sure I eat a supportive breakfast (even though I'm half asleep!). The meals I suggest should take less than four minutes to prepare. If you still think you don't have time in the morning to eat breakfast, then wake up four minutes earlier! Remember, if you skip breakfast you'll slow down your metabolism and compromise your results. Make it a rule to *never* skip breakfast! The serving sizes below are for me. To customize this list for you, remember to use your clenched fist as a guide.

Breakfast

- Three egg whites with one whole egg or one carton of Egg Beaters
  One or two pieces of 100 percent whole or stone wheat bread
  Low fat cheese
  Cottage cheese (1%)
  One tablespoon of flax oil
  Fiber-Psyll

- Oatmeal (whole oats, not instant)
  One scoop protein powder
  Two tablespoons of ground flax seeds (as directed on container)
  Fiber-Psyll

- Two pieces 100 percent whole or stone ground wheat toast
  Three tablespoons of cottage cheese (1%)
  One tablespoon of flax oil
  Fiber-Psyll

- Meal replacement shake
  Mix with two tablespoons of ground flax seeds (as directed on container)
  Fiber-Psyll

Snack between breakfast and lunch or lunch and dinner

- Cottage cheese (1%) with 100 percent whole wheat or flax seed crackers

- Meal replacement shake

- Oatmeal with protein powder

- Egg Beaters (Can be prepared in a microwave at home or work)

- Apple with one tablespoon of peanut butter (no more than once per week)

- Sugar-free Jell-O or pudding

- Chicken breast

Lunch

- Green leafy salad with chicken or tuna. Add cucumbers, tomatoes and cheese for more taste. Use mixture of extra virgin olive oil with flax seed oil (preferred) or some type of reduced calorie dressing

- Chicken, turkey, or fish with brown rice or sweet potato and a green vegetable

- Chicken, turkey, or fish sandwich. Use 100 percent whole or stone ground wheat bread. Add hot sauce, mustard or reduced calorie salad dressing for flavor

- Chicken or tuna roll-ups. Roll strips of chicken or tuna fish in 100 percent whole wheat tortilla shells. Add low-fat cheese, a tomato and a small amount of mayonnaise (light) for taste

- Chicken or Steak Burrito (make yourself—don't buy from a fast-food restaurant!). Chicken or steak strips, low calorie cheese, leafy lettuce, tomato and salsa or hot sauce and whole wheat tortilla shells

Dinner

(Be careful not to overeat, and nothing within three hours of bedtime)

- Green leafy salad with chicken or tuna. Add cucumbers, tomatoes and cheese for more taste. Use mixture of extra virgin olive oil with flax seed oil (preferred) or some type of reduced calorie dressing

- Chicken, turkey, or steak with brown rice or sweet potato and a green vegetable

- Shrimp and chicken kabobs with green peppers, tomatoes and mushrooms

- White fish (orange roughy, haddock or sole) and a sweet potato, grilled

- Ground chicken, turkey or mixed poultry. Add taco seasoning over bed of brown rice or whole grain couscous, or include a whole wheat tortilla and green vegetable

- Steak filet and a sweet potato or whole grain couscous

Grocery List

DAIRY
- ❏ Eggs/Egg Beaters
- ❏ Skim milk
- ❏ Butter
- ❏ Fat free plain yogurt
- ❏ Cottage cheese (1%)
- ❏ Tofu
- ❏ Low fat cheese

MEAT, FISH, POULTRY
- ❏ Chicken (ground or whole)
- ❏ Turkey (ground or whole)
- ❏ Beef
- ❏ Pork
- ❏ Ham (occasionally)
- ❏ Fish (as often as possible)
- ❏ Shellfish
- ❏ Bacon (cheat day)

FRUIT (cheat day)
- ❏ Berries
- ❏ Lemons
- ❏ Limes
- ❏ Oranges
- ❏ Pears
- ❏ Melon
- ❏ Apples

VEGETABLES
- ❏ Broccoli
- ❏ Green beans
- ❏ Cauliflower
- ❏ Celery
- ❏ Cucumbers
- ❏ Garlic
- ❏ Lettuce (leafy)
- ❏ Mushrooms
- ❏ Onions
- ❏ Peppers
- ❏ Sweet potatoes (yams)
- ❏ Spinach
- ❏ Tomatoes
- ❏ Asparagus

BREADS
- ❏ 100% Whole or Stone ground Wheat Bread
- ❏ 100% Whole Wheat Pitas or Tortillas

DRY GOODS
- ❏ Oatmeal (whole oats, not instant)
- ❏ Pasta (whole wheat)
- ❏ Beans, lentils or peas
- ❏ Rice (brown or wild)
- ❏ 100% whole or stone ground wheat crackers
- ❏ Flax crackers

CANNED GOODS
- ❏ Mushrooms
- ❏ Stewed Tomatoes
- ❏ Tuna (white albacore in water)
- ❏ Chicken (in water)

CONDIMENTS
- ❏ Extra virgin olive oil
- ❏ Mayonnaise (low fat)
- ❏ Mustard
- ❏ Relish
- ❏ Salsa
- ❏ Salad dressing (low fat)
- ❏ Hot sauce

BEVERAGES
- ❏ Coffee
- ❏ Tea
- ❏ Soft drinks (sugar free)

BEVERAGES, continued

- ❑ Crystal Light
- ❑ Bottled water
- ❑ Beer (cheat days)
- ❑ Wine (cheat days)

SUPPLEMENTS

- ❑ Protein powder (post-workout shake)
- ❑ Meal replacement shakes
- ❑ Flax seeds or oil/fish oil
- ❑ Fiber (guar gum or Fiber-Psyll)

PART IV

BODY IN MOTION

Anatomy of Major Muscle Groups

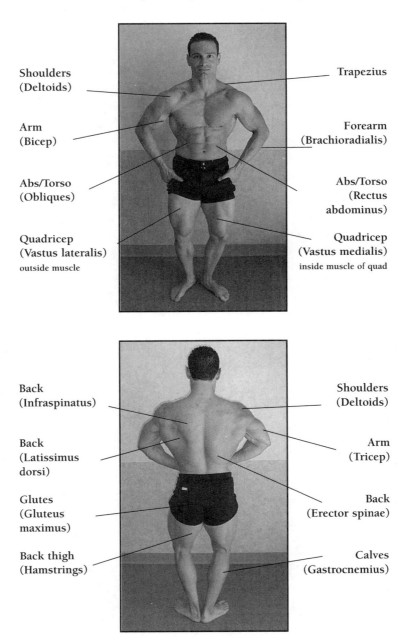

Shoulders
(Deltoids)

Trapezius

Arm
(Bicep)

Forearm
(Brachioradialis)

Abs/Torso
(Obliques)

Abs/Torso
(Rectus
abdominus)

Quadricep
(Vastus lateralis)
outside muscle

Quadricep
(Vastus medialis)
inside muscle of quad

Back
(Infraspinatus)

Shoulders
(Deltoids)

Back
(Latissimus
dorsi)

Arm
(Tricep)

Glutes
(Gluteus
maximus)

Back
(Erector spinae)

Back thigh
(Hamstrings)

Calves
(Gastrocnemius)

These primary muscle groups are the focus of the Lose Fat
Forever system workouts.

18

EXERCISE INSTRUCTIONS

T he following workouts are designed to aid you in beginning a weight-training program. Use the next three sections—The Workouts, A Visual Guide to the Exercises, and Chart Your Progress—in unison. There is nothing "magical" about this or any other workout. You don't need to use this workout program if a personal trainer or some other qualified fitness professional has designed a workout for you. However, I do want you to follow my system of performing three weeks of circuit training, three weeks of endurance training and three weeks of power strength training. Remember, workout variation is absolutely necessary. Also, regardless of the type of resistance training you're doing, I want you to follow my nutritional and cardiovascular advice.

Circuit Training, weeks 1–3

For the first three weeks of the resistance workout, you're going to perform circuit training. Circuit training means that exercises are performed consecutively with little rest between. This is to get the metabolism moving and develop lean muscle tissue. For example, in workout one on page 234, you would begin with the warm-ups, and then the stretches. Perform each stretch twice and hold for twenty seconds. Then perform exercise one, then two, then three, then four, then five, then six. That is set one and a complete circuit. You would then rest for two minutes and perform set two, the same circuit again. Depending on how you feel, you could perform the circuit a total of four times. Write your weights and repetitions next to the exercise name. If necessary, change weight resistance for the exercise(s) before beginning next circuit.

You will notice cardiovascular suggestions below the exercise list. For example, in workout one, the cardiovascular suggestion is to perform fifteen minutes at level five exertion. You can use the treadmill, bike, stair stepper, elliptical machine or walk briskly outside. Don't exceed fifteen minutes to start. Remember, you don't want to exercise away valuable lean muscle tissue. As far as exertion of cardiovascular training, perform at mid-level difficulty. For example, level one would be extremely easy and level ten would be very difficult. Level five means at a good pace, but not too fast. I also recommend that you change your cardiovascular machine often. Don't always use the treadmill or any other machine. For example, walk on the treadmill on Tuesday, ride the stationary bike on Thursday and use the stair stepper on Saturday.

Endurance Training, weeks 4–6

In the fourth week, you will switch to endurance training. Endurance is different than circuit training in that an "endurance interval" is performed twice a set. For example, in workout ten on page 238, you will once again start with the warm-up and stretch, then perform exercise one, the bench press, followed by exercise two, dumbbell chest flys. Exercise three is the endurance interval which can include jump rope, bike, elliptical climber or running. Right after the interval, you would immediately begin exercise four and five, then the sec-

152

ond interval. The endurance interval should be performed at a fast pace for the time allotted, which in workout ten is thirty seconds. The endurance interval is designed to spike your heart rate and condition your body to increase its endurance. Also, your body will produce additional lactic acid as a byproduct of the endurance interval. The additional lactic acid has a metabolic (calorie-burning) effect. So the endurance-training phase focuses on burning fat. After the first circuit or set, rest two minutes and repeat.

If you feel out of breath or light-headed, rest for a longer time or stop. Depending on your fitness level, endurance training may be difficult on your body.

Power Strength Training, weeks 7–9

In week seven on page 243, you will begin power strength training. This phase is designed to increase your strength and lean muscle tissue. Utilizing big muscle groups and performing multi-joint movements, you will create the most amount of heat in the muscle. You will also develop the most amount of lean muscle tissue in this phase. I'm often asked, "Derek, if this phase develops the most lean muscle tissue and burns the most fat, why don't we do it all the time?" The answer is that every workout routine needs to be constantly changed or muscle tissues will no longer be stimulated. Secondly, training too long with multi-joint exercises at a heavy weight and low repetitions can lead to injury. Therefore, you will only perform the power strength-training phase for three weeks at a time. Remember to start with the warm up. When performing power strength training, give yourself one and a half to two minutes between each exercise. Even though the focus of this phase is heavier weight with fewer repetitions, I advise you to start light and add weight as you feel the need to challenge yourself. Utilize www.Alessifit.com for a demonstration of these exercises. Also, this is the phase where a personal trainer will be most valuable. The power strength training exercises are the most difficult to perform and take the longest to learn. A trainer can help you learn these exercises safely and correctly.

After power strength training, the focus of the workout repeats back to circuit training. This time, focus on working the muscles more intensly by adding additional weight or repetitions.

- Weeks 10–12: Circuit training
- Weeks 13–15: Endurance training
- Weeks 16–18: Power strength training

Remember, these workouts are suggestions. I don't want you to get frustrated if these exercises are not available to you or if you find them difficult. If you are discouraged or are having trouble with any part of weight training, please contact a personal trainer for assistance. Don't quit—your results depend upon it!

19

THE WORKOUTS

Week 1

If your workouts get off schedule from what is on the "game plan," just make sure that you're weight training three times per week and doing cardiovascular training six times per week. Refer to chapter 21 to chart your progress and follow the circuit training workout.

Day 1: Circuit training: designed to begin to build lean muscle tissue and get the metabolism moving. You will also perform fifteen minutes of cardiovascular training.

EAT: Lean protein, slow-releasing carbohydrate, and vegetable every three to three and a half hours. Drink a minimum of half your body weight in ounces of water and take a fiber supplement. Drink a meal replacement shake if you won't eat otherwise. Remember your post-workout protein shake.

Grade 1-10 [ ]

Day 2: Ten minutes of cardiovascular training on your own. Make sure that you're moving at a moderate pace (about a level of six to seven on a scale of one to ten). You can walk, bike, stair step, cross-country ski or do any activity where you are moving continuously for at least ten minutes.

EAT: Lean protein, slow-releasing carbohydrate, and vegetable every three to three and a half hours. Drink a minimum of half your body weight in ounces of water and take a fiber supplement. Drink a meal replacement shake if necessary.

Grade 1-10 ☐

Day 3: Circuit training: designed to begin to build lean muscle tissue and get the metabolism moving. You will also perform fifteen minutes of cardiovascular training.

EAT: Lean protein, slow-releasing carbohydrate, and vegetable every three to three and a half hours. Drink a minimum of half your body weight in ounces of water and take a fiber supplement. Drink a meal replacement shake if necessary.

Grade 1-10 ☐

Day 4: Ten minutes of cardiovascular training on your own. Make sure that you're moving at a moderate pace.

EAT: Lean protein, slow-releasing carbohydrate, and vegetable every three to three and a half hours. Drink a minimum of half your body weight in ounces of water and take a fiber supplement. Drink a meal replacement shake if necessary.

Grade 1-10 ☐

Day 5: Circuit training: designed to begin to build lean muscle tissue and get the metabolism moving. You will also perform fifteen minutes of cardiovascular training.

EAT: Lean protein, slow-releasing carbohydrate, and vegetable every three to three and a half hours. Drink a minimum of half your body weight in ounces of water and take a fiber supplement. Drink a meal replacement shake if necessary.

Grade 1-10 ☐

Day 6: Ten minutes of cardiovascular training on your own. Make sure that you're moving at a moderate pace.

EAT: Lean protein, slow-releasing carbohydrate, and vegetable every three to three and a half hours. Drink a minimum of half your body weight in ounces of water and take a fiber supplement. Drink a meal replacement shake if necessary.

Grade 1-10 ☐

156

Day 7: Rest, Cheat Day—Eat whatever you want, in moderation. Remember meal frequency!

Total Score for the Week [ ]

The total score for the week should not be less than 48. If it is, your effort will need to improve to see results!

Week 2

You'll progress with weight training to stimulate an increase in your metabolism and will begin to initiate some shifts in your percentage of body fat.

Day 8: Circuit training: designed to build lean muscle tissue and get the metabolism moving. You will also perform twenty minutes of cardiovascular training.

EAT: Lean protein, slow-releasing carbohydrate, and vegetable every three to three and a half hours. Drink a minimum of half your body weight in ounces of water and take a fiber supplement. Drink a meal replacement shake if necessary. Remember your post-workout protein shake.

Grade 1-10 [ ]

Day 9: Fifteen minutes of cardiovascular training on your own. Make sure that you are moving at a moderate pace.

EAT: Lean protein, slow-releasing carbohydrate, and vegetable every three to three and a half hours. Drink a minimum of half your body weight in ounces of water and take a fiber supplement. Drink a meal replacement shake if necessary.

Grade 1-10 [ ]

Day 10: Circuit training: designed to build lean muscle tissue and get the metabolism moving. You will also perform twenty minutes of cardiovascular training.

EAT: Lean protein, slow-releasing carbohydrate, and vegetable every three to three and a half hours. Drink a minimum of half your body weight in ounces of water and take a fiber supplement. Drink a meal replacement shake if necessary.

Grade 1-10 [ ]

Day 11: Fifteen minutes of cardiovascular training on your own. Make sure that you are moving at a moderate pace.

EAT: Lean protein, slow-releasing carbohydrate, and vegetable every three to three and a half hours. Drink a minimum of half your body weight in ounces of water and take a fiber supplement. Drink a meal replacement shake if necessary.

Grade 1-10 ☐

Day 12: Circuit training: designed to build lean muscle tissue and get the metabolism moving. You will also perform twenty minutes of cardiovascular training.

EAT: Lean protein, slow-releasing carbohydrate, and vegetable every three to three and a half hours. Drink a minimum of half your body weight in ounces of water and take a fiber supplement. Drink a meal replacement shake if necessary.

Grade 1-10 ☐

Day 13: Fifteen minutes of cardiovascular training on your own. Make sure that you are moving at a moderate pace.

EAT: Lean protein, slow-releasing carbohydrate, and vegetable every three to three and a half hours. Drink a minimum of half your body weight in ounces of water and take a fiber supplement. Drink a meal replacement shake if necessary.

Grade 1-10 ☐

Day 14: Rest, Cheat Day—Eat whatever you want, in moderation. Remember meal frequency!

Total Score for the Week ☐

Make sure your score is accurate! You will soon begin to see and feel results.

Week 3

You will once again increase the intensity of your weight training and cardiovascular training. By now, you should be getting conditioned to eating supportively.

Day 15: Last week of circuit training: designed to build lean muscle tissue and get the metabolism moving. You will also perform twenty-five minutes of cardiovascular training.

EAT: Lean protein, slow-releasing carbohydrate, and vegetable every three to three and a half hours. Drink a minimum of half your body weight in ounces of water and take a fiber supplement. Drink a meal replacement shake if necessary. Remember your post-workout protein shake.

Grade 1-10

Day 16: Twenty minutes of cardiovascular training on your own. Make sure that you are moving at a moderate pace.

EAT: Lean protein, slow-releasing carbohydrate, and vegetable every three to three and a half hours. Drink a minimum of half your body weight in ounces of water and take a fiber supplement. Drink a meal replacement shake if necessary.

Grade 1-10

Day 17: Circuit training: designed to build lean muscle tissue and get the metabolism moving. You will also perform twenty-five minutes of cardiovascular training.

EAT: Lean protein, slow-releasing carbohydrate, and vegetable every three to three and a half hours. Drink a minimum of half your body weight in ounces of water and take a fiber supplement. Drink a meal replacement shake if necessary.

Grade 1-10

Day 18: Twenty minutes of cardiovascular training on your own. Make sure that you are moving at a moderate pace.

EAT: Lean protein, slow-releasing carbohydrate, and vegetable every three to three and a half hours. Drink a minimum of half your body weight in ounces of water and take a fiber supplement. Drink a meal replacement shake if necessary.

Grade 1-10

Day 19: Last week of circuit training: designed to build lean muscle tissue and get the metabolism moving. You will also perform twenty-five minutes of cardiovascular training.

EAT: Lean protein, slow-releasing carbohydrate, and vegetable every three to three and a half hours. Drink a minimum

of half your body weight in ounces of water and take a fiber sup-plement. Drink a meal replacement shake if necessary.

Grade 1-10 ☐

Day 20: Twenty minutes of cardiovascular training on your own. Make sure that you are moving at a moderate pace.

EAT: Lean protein, slow-releasing carbohydrate, and veg-etable every three to three and a half hours. Drink a minimum of half your body weight in ounces of water and take a fiber sup-plement. Drink a meal replacement shake if necessary.

Grade 1-10 ☐

Day 21: Rest, Cheat Day—Eat whatever you want, in moderation. Remember meal frequency!

Total Score for the Week ☐

Congratulations! You've made it through the first segment, but don't get on the scale yet! Next we begin endurance train-ing.

Week 4

You will begin endurance training with shortened rest periods. This is designed to keep your heart rate elevated throughout the entire workout. New exercises are added and so is a protein day.

Day 22: Endurance training. Continue to build muscle and get the heart rate moving, baby! You will also perform thirty minutes of cardiovascular training.

EAT: Lean protein, slow-releasing carbohydrate, and veg-etable every three to three and a half hours. Drink a minimum of half your body weight in ounces of water and take a fiber sup-plement. Drink a meal replacement shake if necessary. Remember your post-workout protein shake.

Grade 1-10 ☐

Day 23: Twenty minutes of cardiovascular training on your own. Make sure that you are moving at a moderate pace.

EAT: Protein Day. Lean protein and a vegetable every three to three and a half hours. Consume a minimum of half your body weight in ounces of water and take a fiber supplement. To accelerate fat loss, don't eat carbohydrates on non-weight training days. Eat a larger portion of lean protein and vegetables. Drink a protein shake.

Grade 1-10 ☐

Day 24: Endurance training. Continue to build muscle and get the heart rate moving. You will also perform thirty minutes of cardiovascular training.

EAT: Lean protein, slow-releasing carbohydrate, and vegetable every three to three and a half hours. Drink a minimum of half your body weight in ounces of water and take a fiber supplement. Drink a meal replacement shake if necessary.

Grade 1-10 ☐

Day 25: Twenty minutes of cardiovascular training on your own. Make sure that you are moving at a moderate pace.

EAT: Protein Day. Lean protein and a vegetable every three to three and a half hours. Consume a minimum of half your body weight in ounces of water and take a fiber supplement. Drink a protein shake.

Grade 1-10 ☐

Day 26: Endurance training. Continue to build muscle and get the heart rate moving. You will also perform thirty minutes of cardiovascular training.

EAT: Lean protein, slow-releasing carbohydrate, and vegetable every three to three and a half hours. Drink a minimum of half your body weight in ounces of water and take a fiber supplement. Drink a meal replacement shake if necessary.

Grade 1-10 ☐

Day 27: Twenty minutes of cardiovascular training on your own. Make sure that you are moving at a moderate pace.

EAT: Protein Day. Lean protein and a vegetable every three to three and a half hours. Consume a minimum of half your body weight in ounces of water and take a fiber supplement. Drink a protein shake.

Grade 1-10 ☐

Day 28: Rest, Cheat Day—Eat whatever you want, in moderation. Remember meal frequency!

Total Score for the Week [ ]

You should begin to notice a change in the way your clothes fit. You're losing fat!

Week 5

You will continue endurance training with shortened rest periods. This is designed to keep your heart rate elevated throughout the entire workout.

Day 29: Endurance training. Continue to build muscle and get the heart rate moving. Also, perform thirty minutes of cardiovascular training.

EAT: Lean protein, slow-releasing carbohydrate, and vegetable every three to three and a half hours. Drink a minimum of half your body weight in ounces of water and take a fiber supplement. Drink a meal replacement shake if necessary.

Grade 1-10 [ ]

Day 30: Twenty minutes of cardiovascular training on your own. Make sure that you are moving at a moderate pace.

EAT: Protein Day. Lean protein and a vegetable every three to three and a half hours. Consume a minimum of half your body weight in ounces of water and take a fiber supplement. To accelerate fat loss, don't eat carbohydrates on non-weight training days. Eat a larger portion of lean protein and vegetables. Drink a protein shake.

Grade 1-10 [ ]

Day 31: Endurance training. Continue to build muscle and get the heart rate moving. Also, perform thirty minutes of cardiovascular training.

EAT: Lean protein, slow-releasing carbohydrate, and vegetable every three to three and a half hours. Drink a minimum of half your body weight in ounces of water and take a fiber supplement. Drink a meal replacement shake if necessary.

Grade 1-10 [ ]

Day 32: Twenty minutes of cardiovascular training on your own. Make sure that you are moving at a moderate pace.

EAT: Protein Day. Lean protein and a vegetable every three to three and a half hours. Consume a minimum of half your body weight in ounces of water and take a fiber supplement. Drink a protein shake.

Grade 1-10 ☐

Day 33: Endurance training. Continue to build muscle and get the heart rate moving. Also, perform thirty minutes of cardiovascular training.

EAT: Lean protein, slow-releasing carbohydrate, and vegetable every three to three and a half hours. Drink a minimum of half your body weight in ounces of water and take a fiber supplement. Drink a meal replacement shake if necessary.

Grade 1-10 ☐

Day 34: Twenty minutes of cardiovascular training on your own. Make sure that you are moving at a moderate pace.

EAT: Protein Day. Lean protein and a vegetable every three to three and a half hours. Consume a minimum of half your body weight in ounces of water and take a fiber supplement. Drink a protein shake.

Grade 1-10 ☐

Day 35: Rest, Cheat Day—Eat whatever you want, in moderation. Remember meal frequency!

Total Score for the Week ☐

Remember, your score for the week should be at least 48! If your effort has been good, you'll see the difference in your body.

Week 6

The final week for endurance training. Next week you will begin power strength training.

Day 36: Endurance training. Continue to build muscle and get the heart rate moving. Also, perform thirty minutes of cardiovascular training.

EAT: Lean protein, slow-releasing carbohydrate, and vegetable every three to three and a half hours. Drink a minimum of half your body weight in ounces of water and take a fiber supplement. Drink a meal replacement shake if necessary.

Grade 1-10 ☐

Day 37: Twenty minutes of cardiovascular training on your own. Make sure that you are moving at a moderate pace.

EAT: Protein Day. Lean protein and a vegetable every three to three and a half hours. Consume a minimum of half your body weight in ounces of water and take a fiber supplement. To accelerate fat loss, don't eat carbohydrates on non-weight training days. Eat a larger portion of lean protein and vegetables. Drink a protein shake.

Grade 1-10 ☐

Day 38: Endurance training. Continue to build muscle and get the heart rate moving. Also, perform thirty minutes of cardiovascular training.

EAT: Lean protein, slow-releasing carbohydrate, and vegetable every three to three and a half hours. Drink a minimum of half your body weight in ounces of water and take a fiber supplement. Drink a meal replacement shake if necessary.

Grade 1-10 ☐

Day 39: Twenty minutes of cardiovascular training on your own. Make sure that you are moving at a moderate pace.

EAT: Protein Day. Lean protein and a vegetable every three to three and a half hours. Consume a minimum of half your body weight in ounces of water and take a fiber supplement. Drink a protein shake.

Grade 1-10 ☐

Day 40: Endurance training. Continue to build muscle and get the heart rate moving. Also, perform thirty minutes of cardiovascular training.

EAT: Lean protein, slow-releasing carbohydrate, and vegetable every three to three and a half hours. Drink a minimum of half your body weight in ounces of water and take a fiber supplement. Drink a meal replacement shake if necessary.

Grade 1-10

Day 41: Twenty minutes of cardiovascular training on your own. Make sure that you are moving at a moderate pace.

EAT: Protein Day. Lean protein and a vegetable every three to three and a half hours. Consume a minimum of half your body weight in ounces of water and take a fiber supplement. Drink a protein shake.

Grade 1-10

Day 42: Rest, Cheat Day—Eat whatever you want, in moderation. Remember meal frequency!

Total Score for the Week

Congratulations! You've made it through the second segment. Give yourself a pat on the back, and keep up the good work!

Week 7

Power strength training. Remember, the more muscle you have, the more your metabolism will increase. For the next three weeks you're going to cut back on cardiovascular training because of the increased demand of strength training.

Day 43: Power strength training. Focusing on muscle growth to increase your metabolism. Perform twenty minutes of cardiovascular training.

EAT: Lean protein, slow-releasing carbohydrate, and vegetable every three to three and a half hours. Drink a minimum of half your body weight in ounces of water and take a fiber supplement. Drink a meal replacement shake if necessary.

Grade 1-10

Day 44: Fifteen minutes of cardiovascular training on your own. Make sure that you are moving at a moderate pace.

EAT: Protein Day. Lean protein and a vegetable every three to three and a half hours. Consume a minimum of half your body weight in ounces of water and take a fiber supplement. To accelerate fat loss, don't eat carbohydrates on non-weight training days. Eat a larger portion of lean protein and vegetables. Drink a protein shake.

Grade 1-10 ☐

Day 45: Power strength training. Focusing on muscle growth to increase your metabolism. Perform twenty minutes of cardiovascular training.

EAT: Lean protein, slow-releasing carbohydrate, and vegetable every three to three and a half hours. Drink a minimum of half your body weight in ounces of water and take a fiber supplement. Drink a meal replacement shake if necessary.

Grade 1-10 ☐

Day 46: Fifteen minutes of cardiovascular training on your own. Make sure that you are moving at a moderate pace.

EAT: Protein Day. Lean protein and a vegetable every three to three and a half hours. Consume a minimum of half your body weight in ounces of water and take a fiber supplement. Drink a protein shake.

Grade 1-10 ☐

Day 47: Power strength training. Focusing on muscle growth to increase your metabolism. Perform twenty minutes of cardiovascular training.

EAT: Lean protein, slow-releasing carbohydrate, and vegetable every three to three and a half hours. Drink a minimum of half your body weight in ounces of water and take a fiber supplement. Drink a meal replacement shake if necessary.

Grade 1-10 ☐

Day 48: Fifteen minutes of cardiovascular training on your own. Make sure that you are moving at a moderate pace.

EAT: Protein Day. Lean protein and a vegetable every three to three and a half hours. Consume a minimum of half your body weight in ounces of water and take a fiber supplement. Drink a protein shake.

Grade 1-10

Day 49: Rest, Cheat Day—Eat whatever you want, in moderation. Remember meal frequency!

Total Score for the Week

How do you like power strength training? Your body is continuing to shape, tone and lose fat.

Week 8

Power strength training. For the next two weeks you will continue to cut back on cardiovascular training because of the increased demand of strength training.

Day 50: Power strength training. Focusing on muscle growth to increase your metabolism. Perform twenty minutes of cardiovascular training.

EAT: Lean protein, slow-releasing carbohydrate, and vegetable every three to three and a half hours. Consume a minimum of half your body weight in ounces of water and take a fiber supplement. Drink a meal replacement shake if necessary.

Grade 1-10

Day 51: Fifteen minutes of cardiovascular training on your own. Make sure that you are moving at a moderate pace.

EAT: Protein Day. Lean protein and a vegetable every three to three and a half hours. Consume a minimum of half your body weight in ounces of water and take a fiber supplement. To accelerate fat loss, do not eat carbohydrates on non-weight training days. Eat a larger portion of lean protein and vegetables. Drink a protein shake.

Grade 1-10

Day 52: Power strength training. Focusing on muscle growth to increase your metabolism. Perform twenty minutes of cardiovascular training.

EAT: Lean protein, slow-releasing carbohydrate, and vegetable every three to three and a half hours. Drink a minimum of half your body weight in ounces of water and take a fiber supplement. Drink a meal replacement shake if necessary.

Grade 1-10

Day 53: Fifteen minutes of cardiovascular training on your own. Make sure that you are moving at a moderate pace.

EAT: Protein Day. Lean protein and a vegetable every three to three and a half hours. Consume a minimum of half your body weight in ounces of water and take a fiber supplement. Drink a protein shake.

Grade 1-10

Day 54: Power strength training. Focusing on muscle growth to increase your metabolism. Perform twenty minutes of cardiovascular training.

EAT: Lean protein, slow-releasing carbohydrate, and vegetable every three to three and a half hours. Drink a minimum of half your body weight in ounces of water and take a fiber supplement. Drink a meal replacement shake if necessary.

Grade 1-10

Day 55: Fifteen minutes of cardiovascular training on your own. Make sure that you are moving at a moderate pace.

EAT: Protein Day. Lean protein and a vegetable every three to three and a half hours. Consume a minimum of half your body weight in ounces of water and take a fiber supplement. Drink a protein shake.

Grade 1-10

Day 56: Rest, Cheat Day—Eat whatever you want, in moderation. Remember meal frequency!

Total Score for the Week

Keep gaining strength! One more week of power strength training and we will shift back to circuit training.

Week 9

This is the last week of power strength training. You will continue to build the important lean muscle tissue.

Day 57: Power strength training. Focusing on muscle growth to increase your metabolism. Perform twenty minutes of cardiovascular training.

EAT: Lean protein, slow-releasing carbohydrate, and vegetable every three to three and a half hours. Drink a minimum of half your body weight in ounces of water and take a fiber supplement. Drink a meal replacement shake if necessary.

Grade 1-10 ☐

Day 58: Fifteen minutes of cardiovascular training on your own. Make sure that you are moving at a moderate pace.

EAT: **Protein day.** Lean protein and a vegetable every three to three and a half hours. Drink a minimum of half your body weight in ounces of water and take a fiber supplement. To accelerate fat loss, don't eat carbohydrates on non-weight training days. Eat a larger portion of lean protein and vegetables. Drink a protein shake.

Grade 1-10 ☐

Day 59: Power strength training. Focusing on muscle growth to increase your metabolism. Perform twenty minutes of cardiovascular training.

EAT: Lean protein, slow-releasing carbohydrate, and vegetable every three to three and a half hours. Drink a minimum of half your body weight in ounces of water and take a fiber supplement. Drink a meal replacement shake if necessary.

Grade 1-10 ☐

Day 60: Fifteen minutes of cardiovascular training on your own. Make sure that you are moving at a moderate pace.

EAT: **Protein day.** Lean protein and a vegetable every three to three and a half hours. Drink a minimum of half your body weight in ounces of water and take a fiber supplement. Drink a protein shake.

Grade 1-10 ☐

Day 61: Power strength training. Focusing on muscle growth to increase your metabolism. Perform twenty minutes of cardiovascular training.

EAT: Lean protein, slow-releasing carbohydrate, and vegetable every three to three and a half hours. Drink a minimum of half your body weight in ounces of water and take a fiber supplement. Drink a meal replacement shake if necessary.

Grade 1-10 ☐

Day 62: Fifteen minutes of cardiovascular training on your own. Make sure that you are moving at a moderate pace.

EAT: **Protein day.** Lean protein and a vegetable every three to three and a half hours. Drink a minimum of half your body weight in ounces of water and take a fiber supplement. Drink a protein shake.

Grade 1-10 ☐

Day 63: Rest, Cheat Day—Eat whatever you want, in moderation. Remember meal frequency!

Total Score for the Week ☐

Congratulations! You've made it through the first phase of the system. Now your metabolism should be burning fuel quickly. In the second phase, body fat is going to decrease at a faster pace. Keep up the good work!

Week 10

Remember, if your workouts get off schedule from what is on the "game plan," just make sure that you are weight training three times per week and cardiovascular training six times per week. In order to promote nutritional caloric variation, you are going to eliminate protein day for the next three weeks.

Day 64: Circuit training: designed to build lean muscle tissue and increase the metabolism. Perform twenty-five minutes of cardiovascular training.

EAT: Lean protein, slow-releasing carbohydrate, and vegetable every three to three and a half hours. Drink a minimum of half your body weight in ounces of water and take a fiber supplement. Drink a meal replacement shake if necessary. Remember your post-workout protein shake.

Grade 1-10 ☐

Day 65: Twenty minutes of cardiovascular training on your own. Make sure that you are moving at a moderate pace

EAT: Lean protein, slow-releasing carbohydrate, and vegetable every three to three and a half hours. Drink a minimum of half your body weight in ounces of water and take a fiber supplement. Drink a meal replacement shake if necessary.

Grade 1-10 ☐

Day 66: Perform circuit training and twenty-five minutes of cardiovascular training.

EAT: Lean protein, slow-releasing carbohydrate, and vegetable every three to three and a half hours. Drink a minimum of half your body weight in ounces of water and take a fiber supplement. Drink a meal replacement shake if necessary.

Grade 1-10 ☐

Day 67: Twenty minutes of cardiovascular training on your own. Make sure that you are moving at a moderate pace.

EAT: Lean protein, slow-releasing carbohydrate, and vegetable every three to three and a half hours. Drink a minimum of half your body weight in ounces of water and take a fiber supplement. Drink a meal replacement shake if necessary.

Grade 1-10 ☐

Day 68: Perform circuit training and twenty-five minutes of cardiovascular training.

EAT: Lean protein, slow-releasing carbohydrate, and vegetable every three to three and a half hours. Drink a minimum

of half your body weight in ounces of water and take a fiber supplement. Drink a meal replacement shake if necessary.

Grade 1-10 ☐

Day 69: Twenty minutes of cardiovascular training on your own. Make sure that you are moving at a moderate pace.

EAT: Lean protein, slow-releasing carbohydrate, and vegetable every three to three and a half hours. Drink a minimum of half your body weight in ounces of water and take a fiber supplement. Drink a meal replacement shake if necessary.

Grade 1-10 ☐

Day 70: Rest, Cheat Day—Eat whatever you want, in moderation. Remember meal frequency!

Total Score for the Week ☐

Your total score for the week should not be less than 48.

Week 11

Your body should be conditioned to working out and eating supportively. If you're having trouble, please take the time to reread the book or consult with your trainer.

Day 71: Circuit training: designed to build lean muscle tissue and increase metabolism. Perform twenty-five minutes of cardiovascular training.

EAT: Lean protein, slow-releasing carbohydrate, and vegetable every three to three and a half hours. Drink a minimum of half your body weight in ounces of water and take a fiber supplement. Drink a meal replacement shake if necessary. Remember your post-workout protein shake.

Grade 1-10 ☐

Day 72: Twenty minutes of cardiovascular training on your own. Make sure that you are moving at a moderate pace.

EAT: Lean protein, slow-releasing carbohydrate, and vegetable every three to three and a half hours. Drink a minimum of half your body weight in ounces of water and take a fiber supplement. Drink a meal replacement shake if necessary.

Grade 1-10 ☐

Day 73: Circuit training: designed to build lean muscle tissue and increase metabolism. Perform twenty-five minutes of cardiovascular training.

EAT: Lean protein, slow-releasing carbohydrate, and vegetable every three to three and a half hours. Drink a minimum of half your body weight in ounces of water and take a fiber supplement. Drink a meal replacement shake if necessary.

Grade 1-10

Day 74: Twenty minutes of cardiovascular training on your own. Make sure that you are moving at a moderate pace.

EAT: Lean protein, slow-releasing carbohydrate, and vegetable every three to three and a half hours. Drink a minimum of half your body weight in ounces of water and take a fiber supplement. Drink a meal replacement shake if necessary.

Grade 1-10

Day 75: Circuit training: designed to build lean muscle tissue and increase metabolism. Perform twenty-five minutes of cardiovascular training.

EAT: Lean protein, slow-releasing carbohydrate, and vegetable every three to three and a half hours. Drink a minimum of half your body weight in ounces of water and take a fiber supplement. Drink a meal replacement shake if necessary.

Grade 1-10

Day 76: Twenty minutes of cardiovascular training on your own. Make sure that you are moving at a moderate pace.

EAT: Lean protein, slow-releasing carbohydrate, and vegetable every three to three and a half hours. Drink a minimum of half your body weight in ounces of water and take a fiber supplement. Drink a meal replacement shake if necessary.

Grade 1-10

Day 77: Rest, Cheat Day—Eat whatever you want, in moderation. Remember meal frequency!

Total Score for the Week

Your clothes should fit dramatically different. You're improving your body and the quality of your life!

Week 12

This is the last week of circuit training in this phase. Finish strong!

Day 78: Circuit training: designed to build lean muscle tissue and increase metabolism. Perform twenty-five minutes of cardiovascular training.

EAT: Lean protein, slow-releasing carbohydrate, and vegetable every three to three and a half hours. Drink a minimum of half your body weight in ounces of water and take a fiber supplement. Drink a meal replacement shake if necessary. Remember your post-workout protein shake.

Grade 1-10

Day 79: Twenty minutes of cardiovascular training on your own. Make sure that you are moving at a moderate pace.

EAT: Lean protein, slow-releasing carbohydrate, and vegetable every three to three and a half hours. Drink a minimum of half your body weight in ounces of water and take a fiber supplement. Drink a meal replacement shake if necessary.

Grade 1-10

Day 80: Circuit training: designed to build lean muscle tissue and increase metabolism. Perform twenty-five minutes of cardiovascular training.

EAT: Lean protein, slow-releasing carbohydrate, and vegetable every three to three and a half hours. Drink a minimum of half your body weight in ounces of water and take a fiber supplement. Drink a meal replacement shake if necessary.

Grade 1-10

Day 81: Twenty minutes of cardiovascular training on your own. Make sure that you are moving at a moderate pace.

EAT: Lean protein, slow-releasing carbohydrate, and vegetable every three to three and a half hours. Drink a minimum of half your body weight in ounces of water and take a fiber supplement. Drink a meal replacement shake if necessary.

Grade 1-10

Day 82: Circuit training: designed to build lean muscle tissue and increase metabolism. Perform twenty-five minutes of cardiovascular training.

EAT: Lean protein, slow-releasing carbohydrate, and vegetable every three to three and a half hours. Drink a minimum of half your body weight in ounces of water and take a fiber supplement. Drink a meal replacement shake if necessary.

Grade 1-10

Day 83: Twenty minutes of cardiovascular training on your own. Make sure that you are moving at a moderate pace.

EAT: Lean protein, slow-releasing carbohydrate, and vegetable every three to three and a half hours. Drink a minimum of half your body weight in ounces of water and take a fiber supplement. Drink a meal replacement shake if necessary.

Grade 1-10

Day 84: Rest, Cheat Day—Eat whatever you want, in moderation. Remember meal frequency!

Total Score for the Week

Let's begin to perform endurance training again and really accelerate your results!

Week 13

You will once again perform endurance training with shortened rest periods. New exercises are added and protein day returns for caloric variation to accelerate results.

Day 85: Endurance training. Continue to build muscle and get the heart rate moving! Perform thirty minutes of cardiovascular training.

EAT: Lean protein, slow-releasing carbohydrate, and vegetable every three to three and a half hours. Drink a minimum of half your body weight in ounces of water and take a fiber supplement. Drink a meal replacement shake if necessary.

Grade 1-10

Day 86: Twenty minutes of cardiovascular training on your own. Make sure that you are moving at a moderate pace.

EAT: Protein day. Lean protein and a vegetable every three to three and a half hours. Consume a minimum of half your body weight in ounces of water and take a fiber supplement. To accelerate fat loss, don't eat carbohydrates on non-weight training days. Eat a larger portion of lean protein and vegetables. Drink a protein shake.

Grade 1-10

Day 87: Perform endurance training and thirty minutes of cardiovascular training.

EAT: Lean protein, slow-releasing carbohydrate, and vegetable every three to three and a half hours. Drink a minimum of half your body weight in ounces of water and take a fiber supplement. Drink a meal replacement shake if necessary.

Grade 1-10

Day 88: Twenty minutes of cardiovascular training on your own. Make sure that you are moving at a moderate pace.

EAT: Protein day. Lean protein and a vegetable every three to three and a half hours. Consume a minimum of half your body weight in ounces of water and take a fiber supplement. Drink a protein shake.

Grade 1-10

Day 89: Perform endurance training and thirty minutes of cardiovascular training.

EAT: Lean protein, slow-releasing carbohydrate, and vegetable every three to three and a half hours. Drink a minimum of half your body weight in ounces of water and take a fiber supplement. Drink a meal replacement shake if necessary.

Grade 1-10

Day 90: Twenty minutes of cardiovascular training on your own. Make sure that you are moving at a moderate pace.

EAT: Protein day. Lean protein and a vegetable every three to three and a half hours. Consume a minimum of half your body weight in ounces of water and take a fiber supplement. Drink a protein shake.

Grade 1-10 ☐

Day 91: Rest, Cheat Day—Eat whatever you want, in moderation. Remember meal frequency!

Total Score for the Week ☐

You should begin to notice a big change in your appearance!

Week 14

You will once again perform endurance training with shortened rest periods. Make sure that you're keeping an accurate and honest evaluation of your efforts!

Day 92: Endurance training. Continue to build muscle and get the heart rate moving! Perform thirty minutes of cardiovascular training.

EAT: Lean protein, slow-releasing carbohydrate, and vegetable every three to three and a half hours. Drink a minimum of half your body weight in ounces of water and take a fiber supplement. Drink a meal replacement shake if necessary.

Grade 1-10 ☐

Day 93: Twenty minutes of cardiovascular training on your own. Make sure that you are moving at a moderate pace.

EAT: Protein day. Lean protein and a vegetable every three to three and a half hours. Consume a minimum of half your body weight in ounces of water and take a fiber supplement. To accelerate fat loss, don't eat carbohydrates on non-weight training days. Eat a larger portion of lean protein and vegetables. Drink a protein shake.

Grade 1-10 ☐

Day 94: Endurance training. Continue to build muscle and get the heart rate moving. Perform thirty minutes of cardiovascular training.

EAT: Lean protein, slow-releasing carbohydrate, and vegetable every three to three and a half hours. Drink a minimum of half your body weight in ounces of water and take a fiber supplement. Drink a meal replacement shake if necessary.

Grade 1-10 ☐

Day 95: Twenty minutes of cardiovascular training on your own. Make sure that you are moving at a moderate pace.

EAT: Protein day. Lean protein and a vegetable every three to three and a half hours. Consume a minimum of half your body weight in ounces of water and take a fiber supplement. Drink a protein shake.

Grade 1-10 ☐

Day 96: Endurance training. Continue to build muscle and get the heart rate moving. Perform thirty minutes of cardiovascular training.

EAT: Lean protein, slow-releasing carbohydrate, and vegetable every three to three and a half hours. Drink a minimum of half your body weight in ounces of water and take a fiber supplement. Drink a meal replacement shake if necessary.

Grade 1-10 ☐

Day 97: Twenty minutes of cardiovascular training on your own. Make sure that you are moving at a moderate pace.

EAT: Protein day. Lean protein and a vegetable every three to three and a half hours. Consume a minimum of half your body weight in ounces of water and take a fiber supplement. Drink a protein shake.

Grade 1-10 ☐

Day 98: Rest, Cheat Day—Eat whatever you want, in moderation. Remember meal frequency!

Total Score for the Week ☐

One more week of endurance training and then you are going back to power strength training!

Week 15

Endurance training is performed for the last time in this phase. Your body should be much tighter and more toned than it was fifteen weeks ago. You've kept your commitment!

Day 99: Endurance training. Continue to build muscle and get the heart rate moving! Perform thirty minutes of cardiovascular training.

EAT: Lean protein, slow-releasing carbohydrate, and vegetable every three to three and a half hours. Drink a minimum of half your body weight in ounces of water and take a fiber supplement. Drink a meal replacement shake if necessary.

Grade 1-10

Day 100: Twenty minutes of cardiovascular training on your own. Make sure that you are moving at a moderate pace.

EAT: **Protein day.** Lean protein and a vegetable every three to three and a half hours. Consume a minimum of half your body weight in ounces of water and take a fiber supplement. To accelerate fat loss, don't eat carbohydrates on non-weight training days. Eat a larger portion of lean protein and vegetables. Drink a protein shake.

Grade 1-10

Day 101: Endurance training. Continue to build muscle and get the heart rate moving! Perform thirty minutes of cardiovascular training.

EAT: Lean protein, slow-releasing carbohydrate, and vegetable every three to three and a half hours. Drink a minimum of half your body weight in ounces of water and take a fiber supplement. Drink a meal replacement shake if necessary.

Grade 1-10

Day 102: Twenty minutes of cardiovascular training on your own. Make sure that you are moving at a moderate pace.

EAT: **Protein day.** Lean protein and a vegetable every three to three and a half hours. Consume a minimum of half your body weight in ounces of water and take a fiber supplement. Drink a protein shake.

Grade 1-10 ☐

Day 103: Endurance training. Continue to build muscle and get the heart rate moving! Perform thirty minutes of cardiovascular training.

EAT: Lean protein, slow-releasing carbohydrate, and vegetable every three to three and a half hours. Drink a minimum of half your body weight in ounces of water and take a fiber supplement. Drink a meal replacement shake if necessary.

Grade 1-10 ☐

Day 104: Twenty minutes of cardiovascular training on your own. Make sure that you are moving at a moderate pace.

EAT: Protein day. Lean protein and a vegetable every three to three and a half hours. Consume a minimum of half your body weight in ounces of water and take a fiber supplement. Drink a protein shake.

Grade 1-10 ☐

Day 105: Rest, Cheat Day—Eat whatever you want, in moderation. Remember meal frequency!

Total Score for the Week ☐

Time to power it up again! Three weeks of power strength training are coming up!

Week 16

Power strength training. Remember, the more muscle you have, the faster your metabolism will be. (Relax, you won't look like an Olympic power-lifter!) The next three weeks we are going to cut back on cardiovascular training because of the increased demand of strength training.

Day 106: Power strength training. Focusing on muscle growth to increase your metabolism. Perform twenty minutes of cardiovascular training.

EAT: Lean protein, slow-releasing carbohydrate, and vegetable every three to three and a half hours. Drink a minimum of half your body weight in ounces of water and take a fiber supplement. Drink a meal replacement shake if necessary. Remember your post-workout protein shake.

Grade 1-10

Day 107: Fifteen minutes of cardiovascular training on your own. Make sure that you are moving at a moderate pace.

EAT: Protein day. Lean protein and a vegetable every three to three and a half hours. Consume a minimum of half your body weight in ounces of water and take a fiber supplement. To accelerate fat loss, don't eat carbohydrates on non-weight training days. Eat a larger portion of lean protein and vegetables. Drink a protein shake.

Grade 1-10

Day 108: Perform power strength training and twenty minutes of cardiovascular training

EAT: Lean protein, slow-releasing carbohydrate, and vegetable every three to three and a half hours. Drink a minimum of half your body weight in ounces of water and take a fiber supplement. Drink a meal replacement shake if necessary.

Grade 1-10

Day 109: Fifteen minutes of cardiovascular training on your own. Make sure that you are moving at a moderate pace.

EAT: Protein day. Lean protein and a vegetable every three to three and a half hours. Consume a minimum of half your body weight in ounces of water and take a fiber supplement. Drink a protein shake.

Grade 1-10

Day 110: Perform power strength training and twenty minutes of cardiovascular training.

EAT: Lean protein, slow-releasing carbohydrate, and vegetable every three to three and a half hours. Drink a minimum

of half your body weight in ounces of water and take a fiber supplement. Drink a meal replacement shake if necessary.

Grade 1-10 ☐

Day 111: Fifteen minutes of cardiovascular training on your own. Make sure that you are moving at a moderate pace.

EAT: Protein day. Lean protein and a vegetable every three to three and a half hours. Consume a minimum of half your body weight in ounces of water and take a fiber supplement. Drink a protein shake.

Grade 1-10 ☐

Day 112: Rest, Cheat Day—Eat whatever you want, in moderation. Remember meal frequency!

Total Score for the Week ☐

When you increase your lean muscle tissue, you'll increase your metabolism and burn more fat!

Week 17

Continue power strength training. After next week, we're going to change the entire system and begin phase three. You have performed admirably and kept your commitment. I applaud you!

Day 113: Power strength training. Focusing on muscle growth to increase your metabolism. Perform twenty minutes of cardiovascular training.

EAT: Lean protein, slow-releasing carbohydrate, and vegetable every three to three and a half hours. Drink a minimum of half your body weight in ounces of water and take a fiber supplement. Drink a meal replacement shake if necessary. Remember your post-workout protein shake.

Grade 1-10 ☐

Day 114: Fifteen minutes of cardiovascular training on your own. Make sure that you are moving at a moderate pace.

EAT: Protein day. Lean protein and a vegetable every three to three and a half hours. Drink a minimum of half your body weight in ounces of water and take a fiber supplement. To accelerate fat loss, don't eat carbohydrates on non-weight training days. Eat a larger portion of lean protein and vegetables. Drink a protein shake.

Grade 1-10

Day 115: Perform power strength training and twenty minutes of cardiovascular training

EAT: Lean protein, slow-releasing carbohydrate, and vegetable every three to three and a half hours. Drink a minimum of half your body weight in ounces of water and take a fiber supplement. Drink a meal replacement shake if necessary.

Grade 1-10

Day 116: Fifteen minutes of cardiovascular training on your own. Make sure that you are moving at a moderate pace.

EAT: Protein day. Lean protein and a vegetable every three to three and a half hours. Consume a minimum of half your body weight in ounces of water and take a fiber supplement. Drink a protein shake.

Grade 1-10

Day 117: Perform power strength training and twenty minutes of cardiovascular training

EAT: Lean protein, slow-releasing carbohydrate, and vegetable every three to three and a half hours. Drink a minimum of half your body weight in ounces of water and take a fiber supplement. Drink a meal replacement shake if necessary.

Grade 1-10

Day 118: Fifteen minutes of cardiovascular training on your own. Make sure that you are moving at a moderate pace.

EAT: Protein day. Lean protein and a vegetable every three to three and a half hours. Consume a minimum of half your body weight in ounces of water and take a fiber supplement. Drink a protein shake.

Grade 1-10

Day 119: Rest, Cheat Day—Eat whatever you want, in moderation. Remember meal frequency!

Total Score for the Week

You've worked hard and followed the system well. You should be looking and feeling great!

Week 18

If you are still with me (and I know that only those who truly want to get into better health and fitness are), you have *transformed* your body. You're a different (healthier) person than eighteen weeks ago! You've done wonderfully. I encourage you to keep up the good work!

Day 120: Power strength training. Focusing on muscle growth to increase your metabolism. Perform twenty minutes of cardiovascular training.

EAT: Lean protein, slow-releasing carbohydrate, and vegetable every three to three and a half hours. Drink a minimum of half your body weight in ounces of water and take a fiber supplement. Drink a meal replacement shake if necessary. Remember your post-workout protein shake.

Grade 1-10

Day 121: Fifteen minutes of cardiovascular training on your own. Make sure that you are moving at a moderate pace.

EAT: **Protein day.** Lean protein and a vegetable every three to three and a half hours. Drink a minimum of half your body weight in ounces of water and take a fiber supplement. To accelerate fat loss, don't eat carbohydrates on non-weight training days. Eat a larger portion of lean protein and vegetables. Drink a protein shake.

Grade 1-10

Day 122: Perform power strength training and twenty minutes of cardiovascular training

EAT: Lean protein, slow-releasing carbohydrate, and vegetable every three to three and a half hours. Drink a minimum

of half your body weight in ounces of water and take a fiber supplement. Drink a meal replacement shake if necessary.

Grade 1-10 [　　　]

Day 123: Fifteen minutes of cardiovascular training on your own. Make sure that you are moving at a moderate pace.

EAT: Protein day. Lean protein and a vegetable every three to three and a half hours. Drink a minimum of half your body weight in ounces of water and take a fiber supplement. Drink a protein shake.

Grade 1-10 [　　　]

Day 124: Perform power strength training and twenty minutes of cardiovascular training

EAT: Lean protein, slow-releasing carbohydrate, and vegetable every three to three and a half hours. Drink a minimum of half your body weight in ounces of water and take a fiber supplement. Drink a meal replacement shake if necessary.

Grade 1-10 [　　　]

Day 125: Fifteen minutes of cardiovascular training on your own. Make sure that you are moving at a moderate pace.

EAT: Protein day. Lean protein and a vegetable every three to three and a half hours. Drink a minimum of half your body weight in ounces of water and take a fiber supplement. Drink a protein shake.

Grade 1-10 [　　　]

Day 126: Rest, Cheat Day—Eat whatever you want, in moderation. Remember meal frequency!

Total Score for the Week

Way to finish strong! Good job! Now it is time to set new fitness goals.

20

A VISUAL GUIDE TO THE EXERCISES

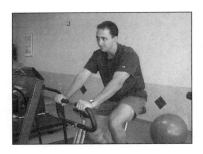

Warm up

Bike-5 minutes, moderate intensity

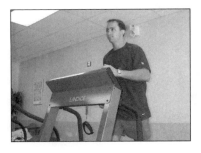

Treadmill-5 minutes, moderate intensity

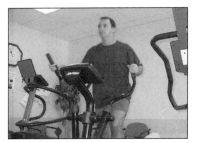

Elliptical climber-5 minutes, moderate intensity

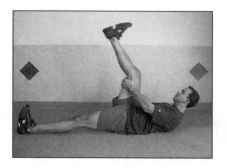

Flexibility

Exercise 1. Hamstring Stretch
Lie on your back. Lift your right leg toward your head. Interlock you hands behind your right knee and keep your left leg flat to the floor. Gradually pull your hamstring until you feel a moderate stretch. Hold 30 seconds. Repeat twice then switch legs.

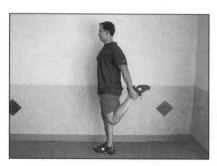

Exercise 2. Lower Back Stretch
Sit on the floor and place your feet double your shoulder width apart. With your knees slightly flexed, lower back straight, and arms extended, reach forward until you feel a stretch in your legs and lower back. Hold for 30 seconds. Repeat twice.

Exercise 3. Quadriceps Stretch
Place your hand against a wall for balance. Bend your right leg towards you buttocks and grab your right ankle. Keep your torso straight and pull tour ankle inward until you feel a stretch in your quadriceps. Hold for 30 seconds. Repeat twice then switch legs.

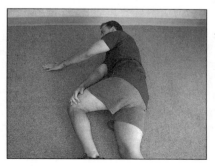

Exercise 4. Lying Shoulder Clock (two pictures)
Lie on the floor on one hip. Rotate your right leg over your left leg. Hold your left arm straight down on the floor.

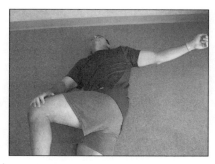

Lying Shoulder Clock,
continued
Start with both hands together at 3'oclock. Glide your right arm counter clockwise while maintaining contact with the floor until it stops near the 9 o'clock position. Your hand will flip over near 12 o'clock. Repeat 10 times than switch sides.

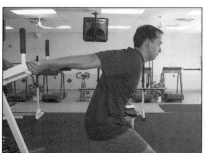

Exercise 5. Shoulder Capsule Stretch
Position your arms on a table or bench. Kneel on one leg and place your arms behind you on bench or table, shoulder width apart. Lean down and away to deepen the shoulder stretch and squeeze your shoulder blades together. Hold for 30 seconds. Repeat twice.

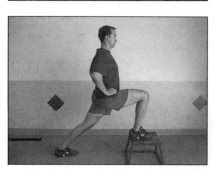

Exercise 6. Psoas (Hip Flexor) Stretch
Place your right leg on a bench or step. Bend your knee at a 90-degree angle and lean forward as far as possible while keeping both feet flat and your left leg straight. Hold the stretch for 30 seconds. Repeat twice then switch legs.

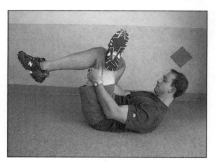

Exercise 7. Gluteus Maximus Stretch
Lie on the floor and bend your right leg at a 90-degree angle and cross over your left leg. Slowly, bend your left leg to a 90-degree angle and interlock your hands behind your left knee. Assist the stretch by pulling with your arms to deepen the stretch. Hold for 30 seconds. Repeat twice then switch legs.

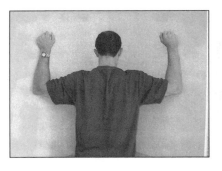

Exercise 8. Standing Chest Stretch

Stand in the corner of the room. No, you are not in trouble yet! Place both of your arms on the opposite walls and bend your elbows at 90 degrees. Slowly, lean forward and simultaneously, pull your shoulder blades together to deepen the stretch. Hold for 30 seconds. Repeat twice.

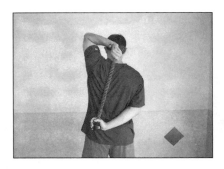

Exercise 9. Triceps Stretch
(two pictures)

Use a towel or a rope. Place your hands about 18 inches apart and behind your back. Pull your bottom hand down and stretch your top hand towards the middle of your back and hold for 30 seconds.

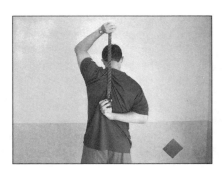

Triceps Stretch, continued

While keeping the same position with your torso and hands, pull your top hand up towards the ceiling and stretch the bottom hand upwards near the middle of your back and hold for 30 seconds. Repeat three times.

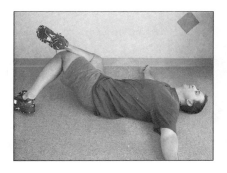

Exercise 10. Quadratus Lumborum Stretch

Lie flat on the floor with your arms on the floor, straight out to your sides. Bend you left knee at 90 degrees and keep your left foot on the floor. Bend your right knee at 90 degrees and position your right ankle over your left knee. With the leverage from your right leg, push your left knee towards the right. Deepen the stretch by going as low as possible. Hold for 30 seconds. Repeat twice and then switch legs.

Abdominals

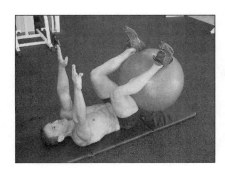

Exercise 1. Ball Crunch Beginning/End
- Position your legs over the Swiss ball, while lying flat on the floor.

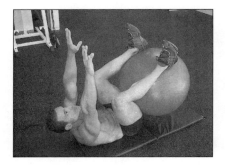

Ball Crunch, Midpoint
- Raise your head and shoulders off the floor 3-4inches, and hold for 2 seconds.
- Exhale as you raise your head and shoulders up; inhale as you return to the floor.

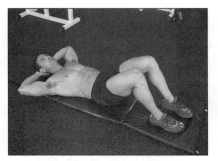

Exercise 2. Sit Ups
Beginning/End
- Begin by lying flat on the floor with your knees bent, feet flat, hands placed at your ears with your elbows back.

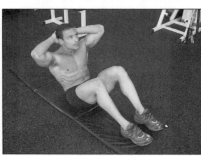

Sit Ups, Midpoint
- Raise your head and shoulders off the floor 3-4 inches while keeping your head in line with your spine. Caution: In order to reduce strain on your neck, do not pull on your head to generate force.
- Exhale as you raise your head and shoulders up; inhale as you return to the floor.

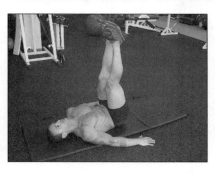

Exercise 3. Hip Extension –Supine
Beginning/End
- Begin by lying flat on the floor with your legs together, straight and pointing up towards the ceiling. Place your arms at a 45-degree angle to your sides for balance and support.

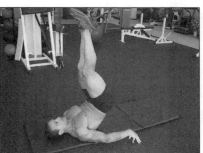

Hip Extension, Midpoint
- Shift your weight to your upper back and extend your hips and butt using your abdominals 2-3 inches off the floor towards the ceiling. Keep your legs straight and moving towards the ceiling.
- Exhale as you raise your hips and butt up, inhale as you return to the floor.

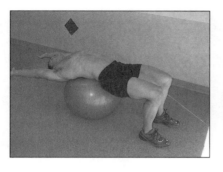

Exercise 4. Swiss Ball Crunches
Beginning/End

- Begin by lying flat on your back on a Swiss ball. Be careful not to roll off the ball. Extend your arms straight back, position your feet shoulder width apart with the majority of your weight resting on your back.

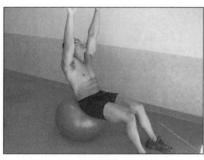

Swiss Ball Crunches, Midpoint

- Without losing your balance, raise your head and shoulders upwards towards the ceiling until your body is seated 90 degrees, straight up on the ball. Keep your arms extended towards the ceiling.
- Exhale as you raise your head and shoulders up; inhale as you return to the floor. (Note: you will feel an initial strain on the front part of your neck. You are not doing the exercise incorrectly. In this initial stage your neck is not strong enough to hold the weight of your head. It will get stronger as you keep performing this exercise.

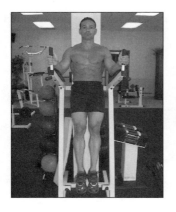

Exercise 5. Vertical Knee Raises Beginning/End

- Begin by using the vertical knee raise bench. Position your body straight, with your elbows and forearms supporting your weight and your feet together.

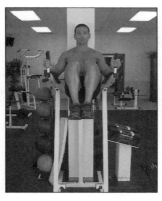

Vertical Knee Raises, Midpoint

- As you balance your weight on your elbows and forearms, lift and bend your knees simultaneously upwards as high as you can using your abdominals. Slowly lower your legs to the beginning position without resting your feet on the foot pegs. Repeat.
- Exhale as you raise your knees up; inhale as you return to the beginning position.

Obliques
(sides of your abs)

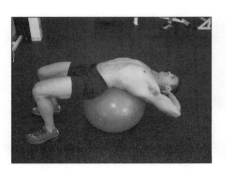

Exercise 1. Swiss Ball Twists
Beginning/End
- Begin by lying flat on your back on a Swiss ball. Be careful not to roll off the ball. Hands placed at your ears with your elbows back, position your feet shoulder width apart with the majority of your weight resting on your back.

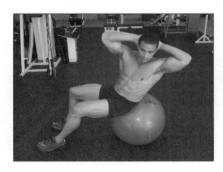

Swiss Ball Twists, Midpoint
- Without losing your balance, raise your head and shoulders upwards towards the ceiling until your reach a 45-degree angle. Begin to rotate your torso, using your abdomen, towards your opposite side. For example, rotate your torso so that your right elbow is moving towards your left knee after you have elevated to 45 degrees. Repeat the same rotational pattern for all repetitions on the same side before you switch and rotate towards the opposite knee.
- Exhale as you raise your head and shoulders up; inhale as you return to the floor. (Note, you will feel an initial strain on the front part of your neck. You are not doing the exercise incorrectly.)

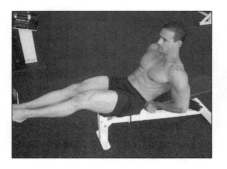

Exercise 2. Twisting Jack Knife
Beginning/End

- Begin by sitting on a flat bench. Place your hands underneath your tailbone and lie back at a 45-degree angle, with your legs placed together and straight.

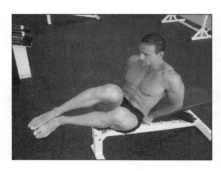

Twisting Jack Knife, Midpoint

- Without moving your upper torso, pull and rotate your knees upwards towards you chest diagonally. For example, your right knee will be pulled towards the left side of your chest. Slowly return your legs to the beginning position. Repeat the same rotational pattern for all repetitions on the same side before you switch and rotate towards the opposite side of your chest.
- Exhale as you raise your knees up; inhale as you return them to the starting position.

Back

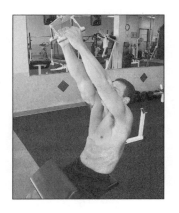

Exercise 1. Lat Pull-Down "Neutral Grip," Beginning/End

- Begin by sitting on a lat pull-down machine. Place your knees underneath the kneepads as to hold you down. Grip the "V" Shaped bar with your hands placed in the middle of each side. Keep your torso erect at a 90-degree angle.

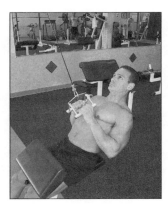

Lat Pull-Down "neutral grip," Midpoint

- Pull the bar down towards the top of your chest using the big muscles of the upper back. As the bar begins to descend, lean your torso back about 10 degrees and arch your back slightly with your chest pushed out. Stop the bar about one inch from your upper chest and pause for one second. Slowly return the bar and your torso to the starting position and allow the weight to stretch your arms and back upward. Repeat.
- Exhale as you pull the bar down towards your body and inhale as you extend your arms up. Remember, when you "exert" you should "exhale." When gravity is pulling the weight naturally, you should "inhale."

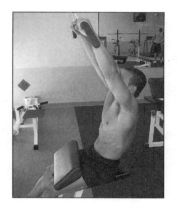

Exercise 2. Lat Pull-Down "Overhand Grip," Beginning/End

- Begin by sitting on a lat pull-down machine. Place your knees underneath the kneepads as to hold you down. Grip the "wide bar" with your hands placed 1 1/2 times your shoulder width, overhand. Keep your torso erect at a 90-degree angle.

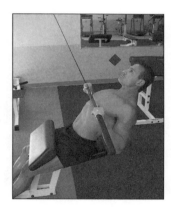

Lat Pull-Down "Overhand Grip," Midpoint

- Pull the bar down towards the top of your chest using the big muscles of the upper back. As the bar begins to descend, lean your torso back about 10 degrees and arch your back slightly with your chest pushed out. Stop the bar about one inch from your upper chest and pause for one second. Slowly return the bar and your torso to the starting position and allow the weight to stretch your arms and back upward. Repeat.
- Exhale as you pull the bar down towards your body and inhale as you extend your arms up.

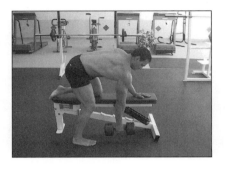

Exercise 3. Dumbbell One Arm Rows
Beginning/End
- Place your left knee and left hand on a flat bench. Position your right foot on the floor and parallel with your left knee. Pick up the dumbbell with your right hand and flatten your back so that there is no curvature of your spine.

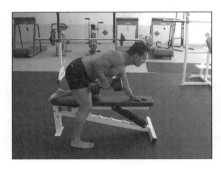

Dumbbell One Arm Rows, Midpoint
- Without rounding your back, pull your right elbow up towards the ceiling. At the top position, the dumbbell should be two inches from your chest. Slowly lower the dumbbell to the starting position and repeat for the entire set using the same arm. After you have performed the desired repetitions, switch arms. Remember, this is a back exercise so focus on initiating the movement using your upper back and not your arms.
- Exhale as you raise your elbow up towards the ceiling; inhale as you return back to the starting position.

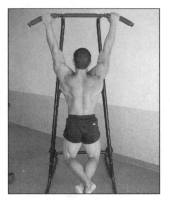

Exercise 4. Pull-ups, Beginning/End

- Begin by using a pull-up/chin-up bar or machine. Grip the bar with your hands placed 1 1/2 times your shoulder width, overhand. Keep your torso erect at a 90-degree angle, cross your feet and bend your knees at 90 degrees.

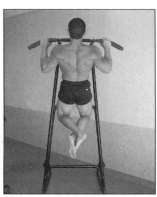

Pull-ups, Midpoint

- Using your upper back, pull yourself up until your chin is just over the bar. Hold the top position for one second and lower yourself down slowly. Do not hit your chin or nose on the bar, it will leave a mark! Repeat.
- Exhale as you pull yourself up; inhale as you lower yourself down.

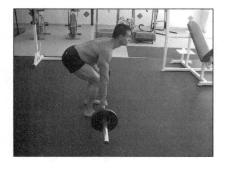

Exercise 5. Barbell Bent Over Row
Beginning/End

- Begin by positioning your feet shoulder width apart, knees slightly flexed and bent over 90 degrees from your waist. Grip the straight bar with an overhand grip, 1 1/2 times your shoulder width apart. Flatten your back so there is no curvature of the spine.

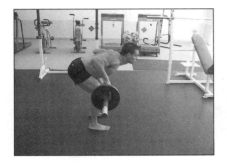

Barbell Bent Over Row, Midpoint

- While maintaining a flat back and your torso bent over at 90 degrees, pull the bar into your chest with your elbows pointing up towards the ceiling. Slowly lower the bar to the beginning position and repeat. It is important to use your back to initiate the movement and not your arms. If you feel pressure or pain in your lower back while performing this exercise, stop and get help from a professional fitness trainer. This exercise is great for keeping you back strong and developing lean muscle tissue, but it must be performed correctly.
- Exhale as you pull the weight up; inhale as you lower the weight back down.

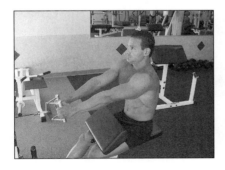

Exercise 6. Seated Cable Row Beginning/End

- Begin by sitting on a seated cable machine. Place your feet straight forward on the footplates. Grip the "V" Shaped bar with your hands placed in the middle of each side. Keep your torso erect at a 90-degree angle.

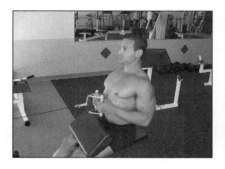

Seated Cable Row, Midpoint
- Pull the bar towards you upper abdomen using the muscles of the mid back. As you pull the bar towards your body, lean your torso back about 10 degrees and arch your back slightly with your chest pushed out. Stop the bar about one inch from your upper abdomen and pause for one second. Slowly return the bar and your torso to the starting position and allow the weight to stretch your arms and back forward. Repeat.
- Exhale as you pull the bar into you body; inhale as you stretch forward.

Upper Back

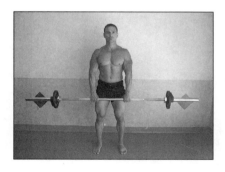

Exercise 1. Upright Rows Beginning/End
- Begin with your feet flat, shoulder width apart. Grip the straight bar overhand with hands placed about 6 inches apart, arms straight.

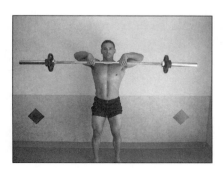

Upright Rows, Midpoint
- Elevate the bar by pulling your elbows upwards towards the ceiling. Do not rock your body. Bring the bar "collar bone" level and pause for one second. Slowly lower the bar using your shoulders until arms are straight. Do not pull the bar into your jaw or teeth. Repeat.
- Exhale as you pull the bar up; inhale as you lower the bar down.

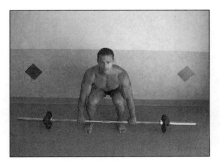

Exercise 2. High Pull, Beginning/End

• Begin with your feet flat, shoulder width apart. Bend you knees and lower your body down to pick up the straight bar off the floor. Grip the bar with an overhand grip, 1 1/2 shoulder widths apart. Make certain there is no curvature of the spine and position your back at a 45-degree angle with your butt down. Keep your head up.

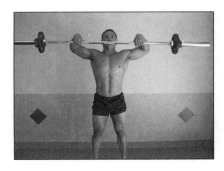

High Pull, Midpoint

• Initially, use your legs to propel the bar up, without stopping the momentum of the bar, continue to pull the bar using your upper back and shoulders until the bar is eye level, elbows slightly bent and the bar is about 4 inches in front of your face. Lower the bar down in one motion to the floor by straightening your arms and bending your legs. After the bar touches the floor, repeat. This is an explosive and complex movement. Initially, practice with a very light weight and get help if you have any questions.

• Exhale as you explode up towards your eyes; inhale as you return the bar to the floor.

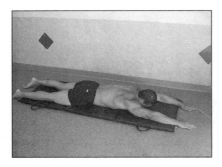

Lower Back

Exercise 1. Superman
Beginning/End
- Begin by lying flat on the floor or mat with your belly and face down. Extend your arms and legs out straight.

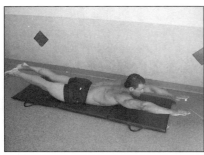

Superman, Midpoint
- Lift your arms, head and legs all simultaneously and shift your weight to your belly. Hold for 3 seconds and slowly return to the floor.
- Exhale as you lift up; inhale as you lower yourself down.

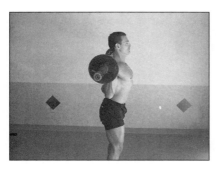

Exercise 2. Good Mornings
Beginning/End
- Begin with the straight bar resting on your shoulders (trapizius). Feet shoulder width apart and torso erect.

Good Mornings, Midpoint
- Flex your knees slightly and by bending at the waist slowly lower your torso between 45 to 90 degrees. Your back should be straight without any curvature of the spine. Push your butt back and try to feel the muscles of your back/hamstring and butt doing the work. Raise yourself back up to the beginning position and repeat.
- Inhale on the way down and exhale on the way back up.

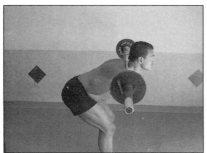

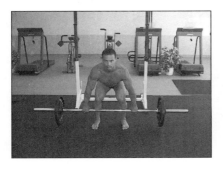

Legs

Exercise 1. Barbell Deadlifts
Beginning/End

- Begin with your feet flat, shoulder width apart. Bend you knees and lower your body down to pick up the straight bar off the floor. Grip the bar with an overhand grip, 1 1/2 shoulder widths apart. Make certain there is no curvature of the spine and position your back at a 45-degree angle with your butt down. Keep your head up

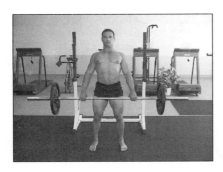

Barbell Deadlifts, Midpoint

- Using your legs, forcefully lift the bar up to your upper thigh. Do not bend your arms. Stand erect and pause for two seconds and return the weight slowly to the floor and repeat. Make sure to use your legs and minimize the pressure on your lower back.
- Exhale on the way up: inhale as you return the bar to the floor.

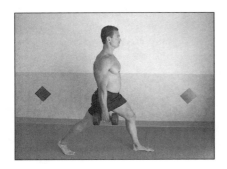

Exercise 2. Dumbbell Split Squats
Beginning/End

- Begin by stepping forward with your right foot. Place equal weight on both of your feet.

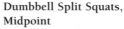

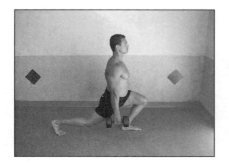

Dumbbell Split Squats, Midpoint

- Bend both of your knees and lower yourself straight down until your left knee is two inches off the floor and your right knee is bent at a 90-degree angle. Pause for one second and push yourself up into the starting position. Repeat. Keep the right foot forward until the end of the set and then switch feet.
- Inhale as you lower your body down and exhale as you push yourself up.

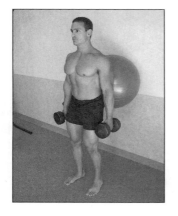

Exercise 3. Swiss Ball Squats Beginning/End

- Begin by placing a Swiss ball against a flat wall. Position the ball between your lower back and the wall. Walk your feet out about one foot in front of your body and shoulder width apart. Lean your weight on the ball and keep your torso erect.

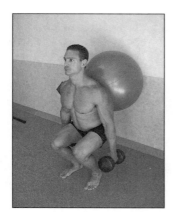

Swiss Ball Squats, Midpoint

- Bend your knees to a 90-degree angle and lower your body down while maintaining a straight upper torso. Let the Swiss ball roll up your back. Keep your head up. Hold the bottom position for one second and press yourself upward, back into the beginning position. Repeat.
- Inhale as you lower your body down: exhale as you push your body up.

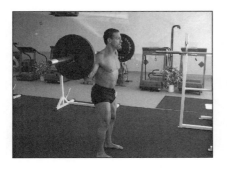

**Exercise 4. Barbell Squats
Beginning/End**
- Begin with the straight bar resting on your shoulders (trapizius). Feet shoulder width apart and torso erect.

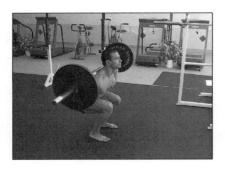

Barbell Squats, Midpoint
- Using your legs, lower your body down and bend your knees to a 90-degree angle. Keep your back straight without any curvature of the spine. Keep your head up. Pause at the bottom for one second and press your body back up to the beginning position. This one of the best leg exercises to perform but it is a complex movement so get help if you have any questions.
- Inhale on the way down; exhale as you push up.

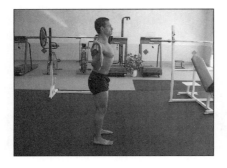

**Exercise 5. Barbell Lunges
Beginning/End**
- Begin with the straight bar resting on your shoulders (trapizius). Feet shoulder width apart and torso erect.

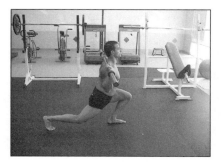

Barbell Lunges, Midpoint
- Begin by stepping forward with your right foot. Bend both of your knees and lower yourself straight down until your left knee is two inches off the floor and your right knee is bent at a 90-degree angle. Keep your head up and lean back. Pause for one second and step backwards into the starting position. Repeat using the same leg until the set is finished. Repeat using the other leg.
- Inhale as you step forward; exhale as you step backwards.

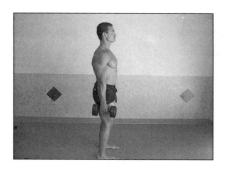

Exercise 6. Dumbbell Lunges
Beginning/End
- Begin by gripping dumbbells in each hand and arms to your sides. Feet shoulder width apart and torso erect.

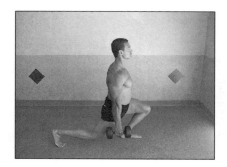

Dumbbell Lunges, Midpoint
- Begin by stepping forward with your right foot. Bend both of your knees and lower yourself straight down until your left knee is two inches off the floor and your right knee is bent at a 90-degree angle. Keep your head up and lean back. Pause for one second and step backwards into the starting position. Repeat using the same leg until the set is finished. Repeat using the other leg.
- Inhale as you step forward; exhale as you step backwards.

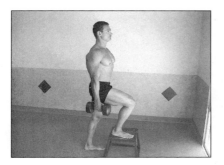

Exercise 7. Dumbbell Step-Ups
Beginning/End

- Begin by placing your right foot squarely on top of a sturdy step or bench. Distribute your weight evenly between both feet. Grip dumbbells in each hand with your arms to your sides. Torso should be erect and head up.

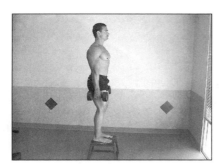

Dumbbell Step-Ups, Midpoint

- Shift your weight to your right foot and step up onto the platform with your left foot, pause on the platform for one second. Keep your torso straight and head up. Carefully, step back down with your left foot and place it on the floor. Keep your right foot on the platform and repeat the movement with your right leg up. After you finish the set, switch and perform with your left leg.
- Exhale as you step up; inhale as you step down to the floor.

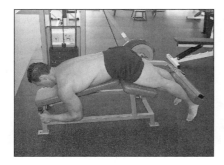

Exercise 8. Hamstring Leg Curl,
Beginning/End

- Begin by lying belly down on a lying leg curl machine. Adjust the ankle plate so that it rests on the back of your ankle and not your calf or feet. Keep your feet straight. Grab the handgrips or hold on to the machine lightly for leverage. Place your knees just off the back of the pad.

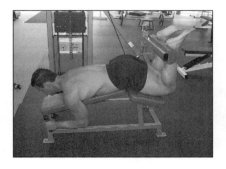

Hamstring Leg Curl, Midpoint
- Curl your legs up and bring your feet as close to your butt as possible without elevating your hips. Keep your head straight and looking down. Hold the top position for one second and lower the weight down slowly to the starting position. Repeat.
- Exhale as you curl the weight up; inhale as you lower the weight to the starting position.

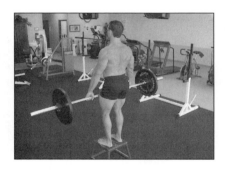

Exercise 9. Barbell Straight Leg Deadlifts, Beginning/End
- Begin by standing on the floor or on a sturdy step. Place your feet flat, shoulder width apart and grab the straight bar with an overhand grip.

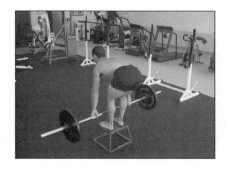

Barbell Straight Leg Deadlifts, Midpoint
- Flex your knees slightly and by bending at the waist slowly lower your torso between 45 to 90 degrees. Your back should be straight without any curvature of the spine. Push your butt back and try to feel the muscles of your back/hamstring and butt doing the work. Raise yourself back up to the beginning position and repeat.
- Inhale on the way down and exhale on the way back up.

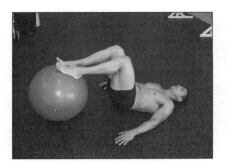

Exercise 10. Swiss Ball Hamstring Bridge, Beginning/End
- Begin by lying flat on your back with your feet placed on top of a Swiss ball. Position your arms to your sides with your hands open for balance.

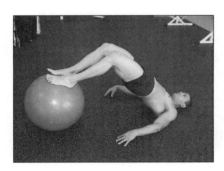

Swiss Ball Hamstring Bridge, Midpoint
- Lift you body off the floor into a "bridge" by placing your weight equally on your upper back and feet. You must balance your feet because the ball may roll. This exercise is good for the hamstrings and glutes and great for developing balance. If it is too difficult at first, put your feet on a bench for more balance.
- Exhale as you raise your body and bridge up; inhale as you lower your body to the floor.

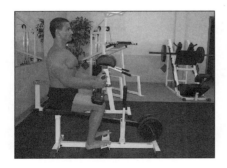

Exercise 11. Seated Calf Raises Beginning/End
- Begin by sitting on a seated calf raise machine. Place your knees comfortably underneath the pad and put the balls of your feet on the footplate. Sit erect at a 90-degree angle with your head forward.

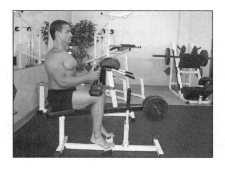

Seated Calf Raises, Midpoint
- Release the lever and slowly lower your heel down as far as you can. Pause at the bottom for one second and press the weight up as high as possible. Hold at the top for one second and lower the weight slowly, stretching the calf. Repeat. Do not rock your torso and keep your head straight.
- Exhale as you raise the weight up; inhale as you lower the weight down.

Chest

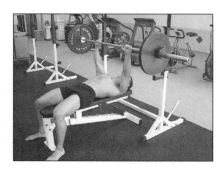

Exercise 1. Barbell Bench Press Beginning/End
- Begin by lying down on a flat bench with your feet flat on the floor. Grip the bar above your head with an overhand grip, a few inches more than shoulder width apart. Lift the bar off the rack and balance it over your chest.

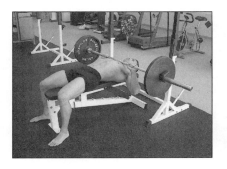

Barbell Bench Press, Midpoint

- Slowly and evenly, lower the bar down to your upper chest. Let the bar touch your chest, but do not let it rest. Immediately, drive the bar off your chest and push straight up until your arms are straight and the bar is directly over your upper chest. Pause at the top for one second and then repeat.
- Inhale as you lower the bar down to your chest: exhale as you press the bar off your chest. (Note: caution should be used when performing this exercise since the weight is above your head, neck and chest. I recommend that you use a spotter or trainer to assist in getting the bar off and on the rack.

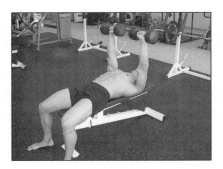

Exercise 2. Dumbbell Chest Press
Beginning/End

- Begin by gripping a dumbbell in each hand and sit on a flat bench. Carefully, lower your body back until you are lying flat on your back with the dumbbells resting on your chest. Raise your arms straight up and position the dumbbell over your chest with your palms facing out. Place your feet flat on the floor.

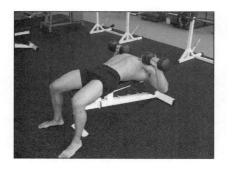

Dumbbell Chest Press, Midpoint

- Slowly lower the dumbbells and bend your arms until the weights are at the side of your chest and parallel to the floor. Your elbows should be pointing towards the floor. Pause at the bottom for one second. Immediately, drive the dumbbells off your chest and push straight up until your arms are straight and the weight is directly over your upper chest. Pause at the top for one second and then repeat.
- Inhale as you lower the bar down to your chest: exhale as you press the weight off your chest.

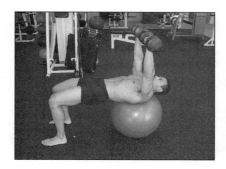

Exercise 3. Dumbbell Swiss Ball Press, Beginning/End

- Begin by gripping a dumbbell in each hand and sit on a Swiss ball. Use caution for the ball can roll. Carefully, lower your body back until you are lying flat on your back with the Swiss ball positioned underneath your shoulder blades and the dumbbells resting on your chest. Raise your arms straight up and position the dumbbell over your chest with your palms facing out. Place your feet flat on the floor.

214

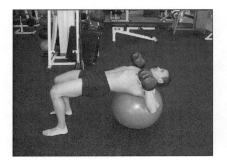

Dumbbell Swiss Ball Press, Midpoint

- Slowly lower the dumbbells and bend your arms until the weights are at the side of your chest and parallel to the floor. Your elbows should be pointing towards the floor. Pause at the bottom for one second. Immediately, drive the dumbbells off your chest and push straight up until your arms are straight and the weight is directly over your upper chest. Pause at the top for one second and then repeat.
- Inhale as you lower the bar down to your chest: exhale as you press the weight off your chest.

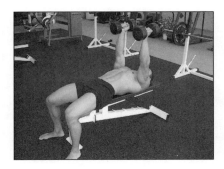

Exercise 4. Dumbbell Chest Fly Beginning/End

- Begin by gripping a dumbbell in each hand and sit on a flat bench. Carefully, lower your body back until you are lying flat on your back with the dumbbells resting on your chest. Raise your arms straight up and position the dumbbell over your chest with your palms facing each other. Place your feet flat on the floor.

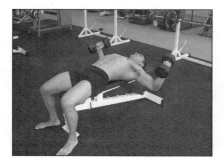

Dumbbell Chest Fly, Midpoint

- Slowly lower the dumbbells and bend your arms until the weights are even with your chest with your palms facing each other. Your arms should be twice your shoulder width apart. Really stretch your chest. Pause at the bottom for one second. Immediately, drive the dumbbells off your chest and push straight up until your arms are straight and the weight is directly over your upper chest. Pause at the top for one second and then repeat.
- Inhale as you lower the weights down to your chest; exhale as you press the weight off your chest.

Exercise 5. Dumbbell Incline Chest Press, Beginning/End

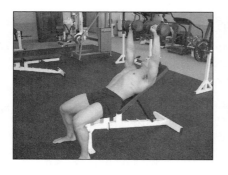

- Begin by gripping a dumbbell in each hand and sit on an incline bench. Carefully, lower your body back until you are lying at a 45-degree angle on the incline bench with the dumbbells resting on your chest. Raise your arms straight up and perpendicular to the floor and position the dumb-bell over your chest with your palms facing out. Place your feet flat on the floor.

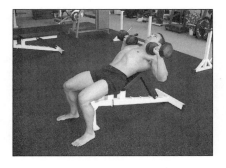

Dumbbell Incline Chest Press, Midpoint

- Slowly lower the dumbbells and bend your arms until the weights are at the side of your chest and parallel to the floor. Your elbows should be pointing towards the floor. Pause at the bottom for one second. Immediately, drive the dumbbells off your chest and push straight up until your arms are straight and the weight is directly over your upper chest. Pause at the top for one second and then repeat. (This exercise is similar to dumbbell chest press, only the angle of the bench has changed.)
- Inhale as you lower the weight down to your chest: exhale as you press the weight off your chest.

Shoulders

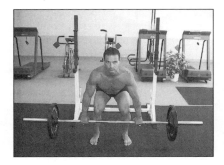

Exercise 1. Barbell Power Cleans
Beginning/End

- Begin with your feet place flat, shoulder width apart. Bend you knees and lower your body down to pick up the straight bar off the floor. Grip the bar with an overhand grip, 1 1/2 shoulder widths apart. Make certain there is no curvature of the spine and position your back at a 45-degree angle with your butt down. Keep your head up.

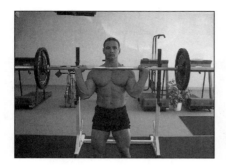

Barbell Power Cleans, Midpoint

• Initially, use your legs to propel the bar up. Without stopping the momentum of the bar, continue to pull the bar using your upper back and shoulders and then rotate the bar towards your body. Your elbows should now be pointing towards the floor and the bar should be level with your collarbone. Lower the bar down in two motions; first to your waist and secondly to the floor by straightening your arms and bending your legs. After the bar touches the floor, repeat. This is an explosive and complex movement. Initially, practice with a very light weight and get help from a personal trainer.

• I don't want you to worry about breathing on this exercise. Just learn the correct form.

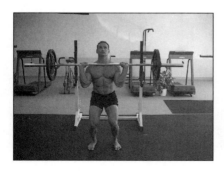

Exercise 2. Barbell Push Press Beginning/End

• Begin with the straight bar at your collar bone using an over handgrip and your hands placed shoulder width apart. Keep your torso erect and flex your knees slightly. Your feet should be flat and even with one another.

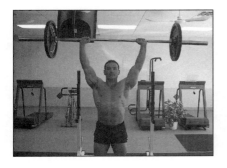

Barbell Push Press, Midpoint

- Bend your knees 45 degrees, while holding the bar collar bone level. Using your legs and shoulders, quickly push the bar straight upward towards the ceiling until your arms are straight and the weight is directly over your head, hold for one second. Slowly lower the bar back down to your collar bone and repeat.
- Exhale as you push the bar over your head; inhale as you lower the bar back down to your collar bone.

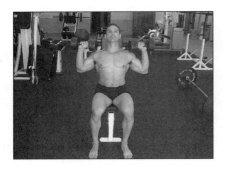

Exercise 3. Dumbbell Shoulder Press
Beginning/End

- Sit on the end of a flat bench or use a shoulder press bench for support and place your upper torso at a 90-degree angle with you feet flat on the floor. Grip a dumbbell in each hand and hold them at shoulder level with you palms facing out and weights parallel to the floor. Keep your head up and look forward into a mirror.

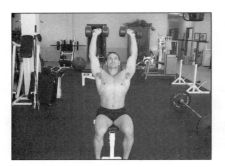

Dumbbell Shoulder Press, Midpoint

- Press the dumbbells up and slightly in and over the top of your head. Your arms should be straight but not locked out. Do not let the dumbbells slam together. Hold for one second. Slowly, lower the weights to the shoulders and repeat.
- Exhale as you press the weights up; inhale as you lower the weight down.

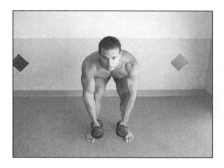

Exercise 4. Dumbbell Rear Lateral Raise, Beginning/End

- Begin by placing your feet shoulder width apart. Grip a dumbbell in each hand and bend over from the waist at 90 degrees so that your upper torso is parallel to the floor. Let your arms hang straight down to your sides with your palms facing each other and keep the weights off the floor. Slightly, bend your knees and keep your back straight.

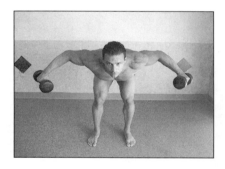

Dumbbell Rear Lateral Raise, Midpoint

- With your elbows slightly bent, start raising your arms upward and to your sides. Try to straighten your arms until they are parallel with the floor. Hold for one second. Slowly lower your arms back down to your sides and repeat. Do not use your legs for momentum or raise your torso during the movement.
- Exhale as you raise your arms up; inhale as you lower the weight down.

Exercise 5. Dumbbell Swiss Ball Shoulder Press, Beginning/End

- Sit on a Swiss ball and place your upper torso at a 90-degree angle with you feet flat on the floor. Grip a dumbbell in each hand and hold them at shoulder level with you palms facing out and weights parallel to the floor. Keep your head up and look forward into a mirror. Use caution when sitting on the Swiss ball so you do not roll off.

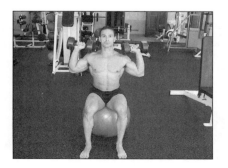

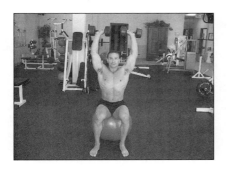

Dumbbell Swiss Ball Shoulder Press, Midpoint
- Press the dumbbells up and slightly in and over the top of your head. Your arms should be straight but not locked out. Do not let the dumbbells slam together. Hold for one second. Slowly, lower the weights to the shoulders and repeat.
- Exhale as you press the weights up; inhale as you lower the weight down.

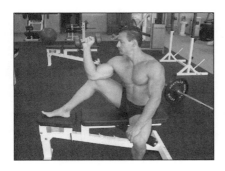

Exercise 6. Dumbbell Rotator Cuff
Beginning/End
- Begin by sitting on a flat bench with you right knee bent and your right foot on the bench. Grip a dumbbell with your right hand and place your right elbow on your right knee with your elbow bent at a 90-degree angle. Your left foot should be on the floor and your left hand resting comfortably.

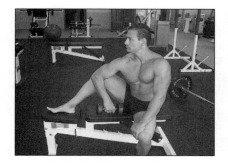

Dumbbell Rotator Cuff, Midpoint

- Slowly begin to inwardly rotate the dumbbell down toward the inside of your leg. Keep your arm and the weight straight. Stretch your internal rotator until you cannot comfortably go any farther. Pause for one second. Begin to change directions and externally rotate the dumbbell back up to the starting position so that your elbow is directly on top of your knee, your arm at a 90-degree angle and the weight pointing towards the ceiling. Pause at the top for one second and repeat.
- Inhale as you internally rotate the weight towards your inner leg; exhale as you externally rotate the weight towards the ceiling.

Biceps

Exercise 1. Dumbbell Standing Hammer Curls, Beginning/End

- Start by standing straight, with your feet shoulder width apart, arms at your sides and grip a dumbbell in each hand, with your palms facing each other.

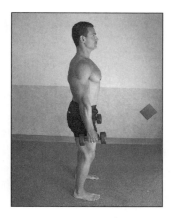

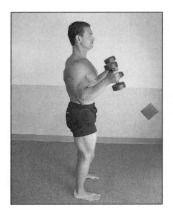

Dumbbell Standing Hammer Curls, Midpoint

- Using your biceps, bend your elbows and curl the weight up until your arms do not go any further. Keep your palms facing each other. Pause at the top for one second. Slowly, lower the weight back down to the starting position and repeat. Do not lean back or rock your body. Any momentum you generate that does not come from your arms will make this exercise ineffective.
- Exhale as you curl the weight up; inhale as you lower the weight down.

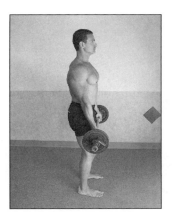

Exercise 2. Barbell or EZ Bar Standing Curls, Beginning/End

- Start by standing straight, with your feet shoulder width apart, arms at your sides and underhand grip either the long straight bar or the EZ curl "curvy" bar with your palms facing out and shoulder width apart.

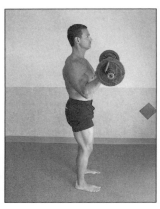

Barbell or EZ Bar Standing Curls, Midpoint

- Using your biceps, bend your elbows and curl the weight up until your arms do not go any further. Pause at the top for one second. Slowly, lower the weight back down to the starting position and repeat.
- Exhale as you curl the weight up; inhale as you lower the weight down.

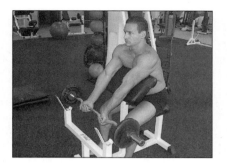

Exercise 3. EZ Bar Preacher Curl
Beginning/End
• Begin by sitting on a preacher bench with your arms resting over the top of the pad, feet flat on the floor and torso straight. Grip the EZ "curvy" bar underhand "palms up" and shoulder width apart.

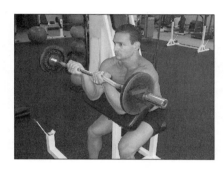

EZ Bar Preacher Curl, Midpoint
• Bend you elbow and using your biceps; curl the weight up as high as you can. Pause at the top for one second and slowly lower the weight down until your arms are straight. Repeat. Do not lean back or rock your body.
• Exhale as you curl the weight up; inhale as you lower the weight down.

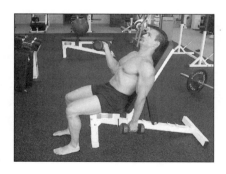

Exercise 4. Dumbbell Seated Alternating Bicep Curls
Beginning/End
• Begin by sitting on an incline bench (45 degree angle). Grip a pair of dumbbells and let your arms hang to your sides with you palms facing each other. Place your feet flat on the floor with your head and back resting on the bench.

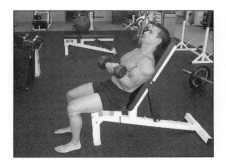

Dumbbell Seated Alternating Bicep Curls, Midpoint

- Curl your right arm up and rotate your hand 90 degrees to the right as you go through the range of motion until your palm is facing the ceiling. Pause at the top for one second and slowly lower the weight down and rotate your hand 90 degrees back to the left as you go through the range of motion, until your hand is facing the other hand. Repeat the same pattern alternating hands.
- Exhale as you curl the weight up; inhale as you lower the weight down.

Triceps

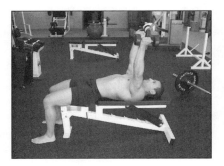

Exercise 1. Dumbbell Lying Tricep Extensions "Skull Crushers"
Beginning/End

- Begin by gripping a dumbbell in each hand and carefully lower yourself to lying down on a flat bench with your back press firmly into the pad. Position your arms straight up and 90 degrees to your torso, with your palms facing each other. Your legs should be bent at 90 degrees and your feet flat on the floor.

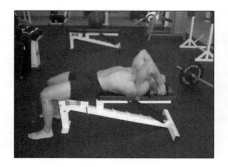

Dumbbell Lying Tricep Extensions "Skull Crushers," Midpoint

• Bend your arms at the elbow and slowly lower the weights to the area near your shoulders and ear. Don't hit yourself in the head! Your upper arms and shoulders should not move. Isolate the movement to your triceps. Pause at the bottom for one second, and then hinge your arms up towards the ceiling until they are straight. Pause at the top for one second then repeat.

• Exhale as you hinge the weight away from your body; inhale as you lower the weight near your body.

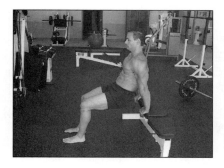

Exercise 2. Bench Dips Beginning/End

• Begin by sitting on the side of a flat bench with you hands placed on the front edge, just outside of your frame. Bend your knees at a 90-degree angle and place your feet shoulder width apart and flat on the floor. Shift your weight just off the bench and support the majority of your weight on your hands. Keep your torso straight and eyes looking forward.

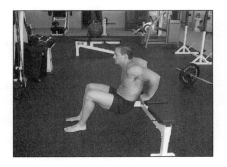

Bench Dips, Midpoint

- Slowly lower your body down by bending your elbows until your upper arm is parallel with the floor. Keep your back straight and close to the bench. Pause at the bottom for one second. Press your body upwards using your triceps until you return back to the starting position. Do not use your hips for momentum. Pause at the top for one second. Repeat. (Note: you can increase then intensity of this exercise by positioning your feet further in front of your body, or by placing a flat weight plate on your thighs.)
- Inhale as you lower your body down; exhale as you press you body up.

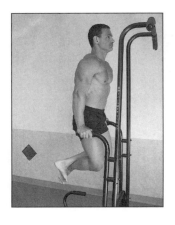

Exercise 3. Dips, Beginning/End

- Begin by placing your hands on the parallel bars of the dip rack. Step or jump up until you are balancing your weight on your hands. Keep your torso straight, head up, knees bent at a 90-degree angle and feet crossed at the ankles.

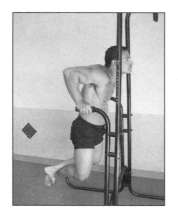

Dips, Midpoint

• Slowly lower your body straight down until your upper arms are parallel with the floor. Pause at the bottom for one second. Press your body back up to the starting position using your triceps. Pause for one second. Repeat. (Note: you can increase the intensity of this exercise by adding weights to a weight belt placed around your waist.) Use a spotter or a personal trainer if you have never performed this exercise before.

• Inhale as you lower your body down; exhale as you press your body up.

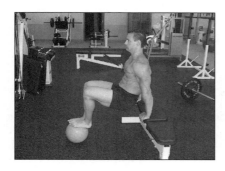

Exercise 4. Bench Dips on Medicine Ball, Beginning/End

• Begin by sitting on the side of a flat bench with you hands placed on the front edge, just outside of your frame. Bend your knees at a 90-degree angle and place your feet on a medicine ball. Shift your weight just off the bench and support the majority of your weight on your hands. Keep your torso straight and eyes looking forward.

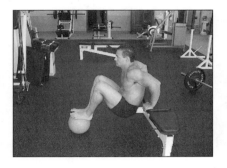

Bench Dips on Medicine Ball, Midpoint

- Slowly lower your body down by bending your elbows until your upper arm is parallel with the floor. Keep your back straight and close to the bench. Pause at the bottom for one second. Press your body upwards using your triceps until you return back to the starting position. Do not use your hips for momentum. Pause at the top for one second. Repeat. (Note: this exercise will work your balance and stability because the medicine ball can roll. Be careful not to fall if the ball rolls.)
- Inhale as you lower your body down; exhale as you press you body up.

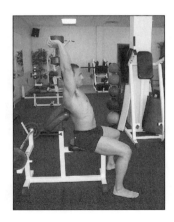

Exercise 5. Dumbbell Seated Tricep Extension, Beginning/End

- Begin by sitting backwards on a preacher bench or at the end of a flat bench. Place your feet shoulder width apart and flat on the floor. Keep your torso straight and head up. Grip one dumbbell and position both of your hands underneath one end of the dumbbell. Straighten your arms above your head and hold the weight vertically with your elbows pointing straight forward.

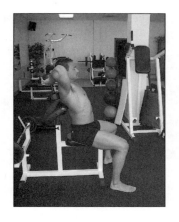

Dumbbell Seated Tricep Extension, Midpoint

• Slowly lower the weight down behind your head by hinging at your elbows until your arms are bent to 90 degrees. Keep your elbows pointing forward and close to your head. Be careful not to hit your head with the weight. Pause at the bottom for one second. Press the weight up using your triceps until your arms are straight overhead. Pause at the top for one second. Repeat.

• Inhale as you lower the weight down; exhale as you press the weight up.

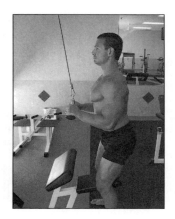

Exercise 6. Tricep Cable Pushdowns
Beginning/End

• Begin by using a high-cable machine. Grip the straight bar overhand, hands placed half your shoulder width apart. Keep your torso and head straight, feet flat on the floor and knees flex slightly. Pull the bar down until your arms are bent at a 90-degree angle at the elbow.

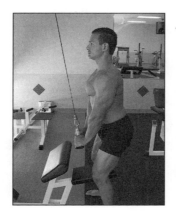

Tricep Cable Pushdowns, Midpoint

- Push the bar down towards the floor in the motion of an arc until you arms are straight and elbows locked. Keep your elbows close to your body. Pause at the bottom for one second. Slowly, hinge your elbows and let the weight return to the starting position. Hold for one second. Repeat. (Note: Do not rock your upper torso forward to generate momentum. Also, keep your head straight throughout the entire range of motion.)
- Exhale as you push your arms down; inhale as you raise you arms back up to the starting position.

21

CHART YOUR PROGRESS

U se these workouts as a guideline. Don't get frustrated if some of these exercises are not available to you, just follow along as best as possible. Remember, for assistance, go to our website www.AlessiFit.com. Always begin with weights you can handle. If a weight is too light, you can always add more. I labeled each exercise by name and number so that you can reference the exercise in the previous section. If you have any questions, check with a personal trainer.

Good luck and don't ever give up!

Week 1—Circuit Training: Get the metabolism moving. Goal: Three weeks of muscle shaping and toning employing a base from which to work. Begin to build lean muscle tissue.

Workout #1

Warm-up:

1. Bike, Treadmill or Elliptical Climber: 5 minutes-Moderate Speed
2. Hamstring Stretch (Flexibility #1)
3. Quadriceps Stretch (Flexibility #3)
4. Gluteus Maximus Stretch (Flexibility #7)

Resistance Exercises

1. Perform 2 circuits of 12 to 15 repetitions.
2. Ball Squats (Legs #3)
3. Hamstring Leg Curl (Legs #8)
4. Dumbbell Chest Press (Chest #2)
5. Lat Pull-Down "Overhand Grip" (Back #2)
6. Superman (Lower Back #1)
7. Ball Crunch (Abs #1)

Cardiovascular: 15 Minutes, Level 5 exertion.

Workout #2

Warm-up:

1. Bike, Treadmill or Elliptical Climber: 5 minutes-Moderate Speed
2. Hamstring Stretch (Flexibility #1)
3 Quadriceps Stretch (Flexibility #3)
4. Gluteus Maximus Stretch (Flexibility #7)

Resistance Exercises

Perform 2 circuits of 12 to 15 repetitions.
1. Dumbbell Shoulder Press (Shoulders #3)
2. Dumbbell Seated Alternating Bicep Curls (Biceps #4)
3. Dumbbell Lying Tricep Extension "Skull Crushers" (Triceps #1)
4. Superman (Lower Back #1)
5. Ball Crunch (Abs #1)
6. Swiss Ball Twists (Obliques #1)

Cardiovascular: 15 Minutes, Level 5 exertion.

Workout #3

Warm-up:

1. Bike, Treadmill or Elliptical Climber: 5 minutes-Moderate Speed
2. Hamstring Stretch (Flexibility #1)
3. Quadriceps Stretch (Flexibility #3)
4. Gluteus Maximus Stretch (Flexibility #7)

Resistance Exercises

Perform 2 circuits of 12 to 15 repetitions.
1. Ball Squats (Legs #3)
2. Hamstring Leg Curl (Legs #8)
3. Dumbbell Chest Press (Chest #2)
4. Lat Pull-Down "Overhand Grip" (Back #2)
5. Superman (Lower Back #1)
6. Ball Crunch (Abs #1)

Cardiovascular: 15 Minutes, Level 5 exertion.

Week 2—Circuit Training, continued. Goal: Continue to build lean muscle tissue to help speed up metabolism. Add resistance if you can while maintaining proper form.

Workout #4

Warm-up:

1. Bike, Treadmill or Elliptical Climber: 5 minutes-Moderate Speed
2. Hamstring Stretch (Flexibility #1)
3. Psaos Stretch (Flexibility #6)
4. Lower Back Stretch (Flexibility #2)

Resistance Exercises

Perform 3 circuits of 12 to 15 repetitions.
1 Dumbbell Shoulder Press (Shoulders #3)
2 Dumbbell Seated Alternating Bicep Curls (Biceps #4)
3 Dumbbell Lying Tricep Extension "Skull Crushers" (Triceps #1)
4 Superman (Lower Back #1)
5 SwissBall Crunches (Abs #4)
6 Swiss Ball Twists (Obliques #1)

Cardiovascular: 20 Minutes, Level 5 exertion.

Workout #5

Warm-up:

1. Bike, Treadmill or Elliptical Climber: 5 minutes-Moderate Speed
2. Hamstring Stretch (Flexibility #1)
3. Quadriceps Stretch (Flexibility #3)
4. Gluteus Maximus Stretch (Flexibility #7)

Resistance Exercises

Perform 3 circuits of 12 to 15 repetitions.
1. Ball Squats (Legs #3)
2. Hamstring Leg Curl (Legs #8)
3. Dumbbell Chest Press (Chest #2)
4. Lat Pull-Down "Overhand Grip" (Back #2)
5. Superman (Lower Back #1)
6. Ball Crunch (Abs #1)

Cardiovascular: 20 Minutes, Level 5 exertion.

Workout #6

Warm-up:

1. Bike, Treadmill or Elliptical Climber: 5 minutes-Moderate Speed
2. Hamstring Stretch (Flexibility #1)
3. Psaos Stretch (Flexibility #6)
4. Lower Back Stretch (Flexibility #2)

Resistance Exercises

Perform 3 circuits of 12 to 15 repetitions.
1. Dumbbell Shoulder Press (Shoulders #3)
2. Dumbbell Seated Alternating Bicep Curls (Biceps #4)
3. Dumbbell Lying Tricep Extension "Skull Crushers" (Triceps #1)
4. Dumbbell Rotator Cuff (Shoulders #6)
5. Superman (Lower Back #1)
6. SwissBall Crunches (Abs #4)
7. Swiss Ball Twists (Obliques #1)

Cardiovascular: 20 Minutes, Level 5 exertion.

Week 3—Last week of beginning phase. Circuit Training, continued. Add resistance if you can while maintaining proper form.

Workout #7

Warm-up:

1. Bike, Treadmill or Elliptical Climber: 5 minutes-Moderate Speed
2. Lower Back Stretch (Flexibility #2)
3. Standing Chest Stretch (Flexibility #8)
4. Gluteus Maximus Stretch (Flexibility #7)

Resistance Exercises

Perform 3 circuits of 12 to 15 repetitions.
1. Dumbbell Split Squats (Legs #2)
2. Barbell Good Mornings (Lower Back #2)
3. Hamstring Leg Curls (Legs #8)
4. Barbell Bench Press (Chest #1)
5. Lat Pull-Down "Overhand Grip" (Back #2)
6. Swiss Ball Crunches (Abs #4)

Cardiovascular: 25 Minutes, Level 6 exertion.

Workout #8

Warm-up:

1. Bike, Treadmill or Elliptical Climber: 5 minutes-Moderate Speed
2. Hamstring Stretch (Flexibility #1)
3. Psaos Stretch (Flexibility #6)
4. Lower Back Stretch (Flexibility #2)

Resistance Exercises

Perform 3 circuits of 12 to 15 repetitions.
1. Dumbbell Shoulder Press (Shoulders #3)
2. Dumbbell Lying Tricep Extension "Skull Crushers" (Triceps #1)
3. Dumbbell Rotator Cuff (Shoulders #6)
4. Dumbbell Standing Hammer Curls (Biceps #1)
5 Superman (Lower Back #1)
6 Swiss Ball Twists (Obliques #1)

Cardiovascular: 25 Minutes, Level 5 exertion.

Workout #9

Warm-up:

1. Bike, Treadmill or Elliptical Climber: 5 minutes-Moderate Speed
2. Lower Back Stretch (Flexibility #2)
3. Standing Chest Stretch (Flexibility #8)
4. Gluteus Maximus Stretch (Flexibility #7)

Resistance Exercises

Perform 3 circuits of 12 to 15 repetitions.
1. Dumbbell Split Squats (Legs #2)
2. Barbell Good Mornings (Lower Back #2)
3. Hamstring Leg Curls (Legs #8)
4. Barbell Bench Press (Chest #1)
5. Lat Pull-Down "Overhand Grip" (Back #2)
6. Seated or Standing Calf Raises (Legs #11)
7. Swiss Ball Crunches (Abs #4)

Cardiovascular: 25 Minutes, Level 6 exertion.

Congratulations! You have made it through the first segment. This is a victory! Your body is using fuel and burning fat more efficiently.

Week 4—Endurance (Interval) Training. Now the body is beginning to burn fat. Goal: Three weeks of endurance training with shortened rest periods. This will ensure that the metabolism speeds up. The "interval" is now introduced into the workout.

Workout #10

Warm-up:

1. Bike, Treadmill or Elliptical Climber: 5 minutes-Moderate Speed
2. Lower Back Stretch (Flexibility #2)
3. Psaos Stretch (Flexibility #6)
4. Shoulder Capsule Stretch (Flexibility #5)

Resistance Exercises

Perform 3 circuits of 12 to 15 repetitions.

1. Barbell Bench Press (Chest #1)
2. Dumbbell Chest Fly (Chest #4)
3. Interval- Bike/Elliptical/Jump Rope- 30 seconds, fast pace
4. Seated Cable Row (Back #6)
5. Lat Pull-Down "Narrow Grip" (Back #1)
6. Interval- Bike/Elliptical/Jump Rope- 30 seconds, fast pace

Cardiovascular: 30 Minutes, Level 7 exertion

Workout #11

Warm-up:

1. Bike, Treadmill or Elliptical Climber: 5 minutes-Moderate Speed
2. Quadratus Lumborum Stretch (Flexibility #10)
3. Hamstring Stretch (Flexibility #1)
4. Shoulder Capsule Stretch (Flexibility #5)

Resistance Exercises

Perform 3 circuits of 12 to 15 repetitions.

1. Dumbbell Step-Ups (Legs #7)
2. Hamstring Leg Curl (Legs #8)
3. Interval- Bike/Elliptical/Jump Rope- 30 seconds, fast pace
4. Swiss Ball Hamstring Bridge (Legs #10)
5. Seated or Standing Calf Raises (Legs #11)
6. Interval- Bike/Elliptical/Jump Rope- 30 seconds, fast pace
7. Twisting Jack Knife (Obliques #2)

Cardiovascular: 30 Minutes, Level 7 exertion

Workout #12

Warm-up:

1. Bike, Treadmill or Elliptical Climber: 5 minutes-Moderate Speed
2. Tricep Stretch (Flexibility #9)
3. Psaos Stretch (Flexibility #6)
4. Shoulder Capsule Stretch (Flexibility #5)

Resistance Exercises

Perform 3 circuits of 12 to 15 repetitions.
1. Barbell Upright Row (Upper Back #1)
2. Barbell or EZ Bar Standing Bicep Curls (Biceps #2) The EZ bar is the "curvy" bar
3. Interval- Bike/Elliptical/Jump Rope- 30 seconds, fast pace
4. Dumbbell Lying Tricep Extension "Skull Crushers" (Triceps #1)
5. Dumbbell Rotator Cuff (Shoulders #6)
6. Interval- Bike/Elliptical/Jump Rope- 30 seconds, fast pace

Cardiovascular: 30 Minutes, Level 7 exertion

Week 5—Endurance (Interval) Training, continued. Add resistance if you can while maintaining proper form.

Workout #13

Warm-up:

1. Bike, Treadmill or Elliptical Climber: 5 minutes-Moderate Speed
2. Lower Back Stretch (Flexibility #2)
3. Psaos Stretch (Flexibility #6)
4. Shoulder Capsule Stretch (Flexibility #5)

Resistance Exercises

Perform 3 circuits of 12 to 15 repetitions.
1. Barbell Bench Press (Chest #1)
2. Dumbbell Chest Fly (Chest #4)
3. Interval- Bike/Elliptical/Jump Rope- 30 seconds, fast pace
4. Seated Cable Row (Back #6)
5. Lat Pull-Down "Narrow Grip" (Back #1)
6. Interval- Bike/Elliptical/Jump Rope- 30 seconds, fast pace

Cardiovascular: 30 Minutes, Level 7 exertion

Workout #14

Warm-up:

1. Bike, Treadmill or Elliptical Climber: 5 minutes-Moderate Speed
2. Quadratus Lumborum Stretch (Flexibility #10)
3. Hamstring Stretch (Flexibility #1)
4. Shoulder Capsule Stretch (Flexibility #5)

Resistance Exercises

Perform 3 circuits of 12 to 15 repetitions.
1. Dumbbell Step-Ups (Legs #7)
2. Hamstring Leg Curl (Legs #8)
3. Interval- Bike/Elliptical/Jump Rope- 30 seconds, fast pace
4. Swiss Ball Hamstring Bridge (Legs #10)
5. Seated or Standing Calf Raises (Legs #11)
6. Interval- Bike/Elliptical/Jump Rope- 30 seconds, fast pace
7. Twisting Jack Knife (Obliques #2)

Cardiovascular: 30 Minutes, Level 7 exertion

Workout #15

Warm-up:

1 Bike, Treadmill or Elliptical Climber: 5 minutes-Moderate Speed
2. Tricep Stretch (Flexibility #9)
3. Psaos Stretch (Flexibility #6)
4. Shoulder Capsule Stretch (Flexibility #5)

Resistance Exercises

Perform 3 circuits of 12 to 15 repetitions.
1. Barbell Upright Row (Upper Back #1)
2. Barbell or EZ Bar "curvy" Standing Bicep Curls (Biceps #2)
3. Interval- Bike/Elliptical/Jump Rope- 30 seconds, fast pace
4. Dumbbell Lying Tricep Extension "Skull Crushers" (Triceps #1)
5. Dumbbell Rotator Cuff (Shoulders #6)
6. Interval- Bike/Elliptical/Jump Rope- 30 seconds, fast pace

Cardiovascular: 30 Minutes, Level 7 exertion

Week 6—Endurance (Interval) Training, Continued. Add resistance if you can while maintaining proper form.

Workout #16

Warm-up:

1. Bike, Treadmill or Elliptical Climber: 5 minutes-Moderate Speed
2. Lower Back Stretch (Flexibility #2)
3. Psaos Stretch (Flexibility #6)
4. Shoulder Capsule Stretch (Flexibility #5)

Resistance Exercises

Perform 3 circuits of 12 to 15 repetitions.

1. Barbell Bench Press (Chest #1)
2. Dumbbell Chest Fly (Chest #4)
3. Interval- Bike/Elliptical/Jump Rope- 30 seconds, fast pace
4. Seated Cable Row (Back #6)
5. Lat Pull-Down "Narrow Grip" (Back #1)
6. Interval- Bike/Elliptical/Jump Rope- 30 seconds, fast pace

Cardiovascular: 30 Minutes, Level 7 exertion

Workout #17

Warm-up:

1. Bike, Treadmill or Elliptical Climber: 5 minutes-Moderate Speed
2. Quadratus Lumborum Stretch (Flexibility #10)
3. Hamstring Stretch (Flexibility #1)
4. Shoulder Capsule Stretch (Flexibility #5)

Resistance Exercises

Perform 3 circuits of 12 to 15 repetitions.

1. Dumbbell Step-Ups (Legs #7)
2. Hamstring Leg Curl (Legs #8)
3. Interval- Bike/Elliptical/Jump Rope- 30 seconds, fast pace
4. Swiss Ball Hamstring Bridge (Legs #10)
5. Seated or Standing Calf Raises (Legs #11)
6. Interval- Bike/Elliptical/Jump Rope- 30 seconds, fast pace
7. Twisting Jack Knife (Obliques #2)

Cardiovascular: 30 Minutes, Level 7 exertion

Workout #18

Warm-up:

1. Bike, Treadmill or Elliptical Climber: 5 minutes-Moderate Speed
2. Tricep Stretch (Flexibility #9)
3. Psaos Stretch (Flexibility #6)
4. Shoulder Capsule Stretch (Flexibility #5)

Resistance Exercises

Perform 3 circuits of 12 to 15 repetitions.

1. Barbell Upright Row (Upper Back #1)
2. Barbell or EZ "curvy" Bar Standing Bicep Curls (Biceps #2)
3. Interval- Bike/Elliptical/Jump Rope- 30 seconds, fast pace
4. Dumbbell Lying Tricep Extension "Skull Crushers" (Triceps #1)
5. Dumbbell Rotator Cuff (Shoulders #6)
6. Interval- Bike/Elliptical/Jump Rope- 30 seconds, fast pace

Cardiovascular: 30 Minutes, Level 7 exertion

Congratulations! You have made it through the second segment, Endurance (Interval) Training. Provided your nutrition is disciplined, you are losing body fat!

Week 7—Power Strength Training. Goal: Three weeks of strength training focusing on muscle growth. Remember, the more muscle you have, the more fat you will burn. Women, don't be worried. You will not look like Zena, the muscle chick!

Workout #19

Warm-up:

1. Bike, Treadmill or Elliptical Climber: 5 minutes-Moderate Speed
2. Hamstring Stretch (Flexibility #1)
3. Lower Back Stretch (Flexibility #2)
4. Shoulder Capsule Stretch (Flexibility #5)

Resistance Exercises

Perform the same exercise <u>3 consecutive times</u>, 8 to 10 reps. Do not circuit train with power exercises.

1. Barbell Power Cleans (Shoulders #1)
2. Barbell Good Mornings (Lower Back #2)
3. Barbell Bench Press (Chest #1)
4. Pullups (Back #4) or Lat-Pulldown Overhand grip (Back #2)
5. Ball Sit up (Abs #4)

Cardiovascular: 20 Minutes, Level 8 exertion

Workout #20

Warm-up:

1. Bike, Treadmill or Elliptical Climber: 5 minutes-Moderate Speed
2. Hamstring Stretch (Flexibility #1)
3. Quadriceps Stretch (Flexibility #3)
4. Gluteus Maximus Stretch (Flexibility #7)

Resistance Exercises

Perform the same exercise <u>3 consecutive times</u>, 8 to 10 reps. Do not circuit train with power exercises.

1. Barbell Deadlifts (Legs #1)
2. Barbell Squats (Legs #4)
3. Barbell Straight Leg Deadlifts (Legs #9)
4. Seated or Standing Calves (Legs #11)

Cardiovascular: 20 Minutes, Level 8 exertion

Workout #21

Warm-up:

1. Bike, Treadmill or Elliptical Climber: 5 minutes-Moderate Speed
2. Quadratus Lumborum Stretch (Flexibility #10)
3. Lying Shoulder Clock (Flexibility #4)
4. Triceps Stretch (Flexibility #9)

Resistance Exercises

Perform the same exercise <u>3 consecutive times</u>, 8 to 10 reps. Do not circuit train with power exercises.

1. Barbell High Pull (Upper back #2)
2. Dumbbell Rotator Cuff (Shoulders #6)
3. Dips (Triceps #3) or Bench Dips (Triceps #2)
4. Barbell or EZ "curvy" Bar Standing (Biceps #2)
5. Vertical Knee Raise (Abs #5)

Cardiovascular: 20 Minutes, Level 8 exertion

Week 8—Power Strength Training, continued.

Workout #22

Warm-up:

1. Bike, Treadmill or Elliptical Climber: 5 minutes-Moderate Speed
2. Hamstring Stretch (Flexibility #1)
3. Lower Back Stretch (Flexibility #2)
4. Shoulder Capsule Stretch (Flexibility #5)

Resistance Exercises

Perform the same exercise 3 consecutive times, 8 to 10 reps. Do not circuit train with power exercises.

1. Barbell Power Cleans (Shoulders #1)
2. Barbell Good Mornings (Lower Back #2)
3. Barbell Bench Press (Chest #1)
4. Pullups (Back #4) or Lat-Pulldown Overhand grip (Back #2)
5. Ball Sit up (Abs #4)

Cardiovascular: 20 Minutes, Level 8 exertion

Workout #23

Warm-up:

1. Bike, Treadmill or Elliptical Climber: 5 minutes-Moderate Speed
2. Hamstring Stretch (Flexibility #1)
3. Quadriceps Stretch (Flexibility #3)
4. Gluteus Maximus Stretch (Flexibility #7)

Resistance Exercises

Perform the same exercise 3 consecutive times, 8 to 10 reps. Do not circuit train with power exercises.

1. Barbell Deadlifts (Legs #1)
2. Barbell Squats (Legs #4)
3. Barbell Straight Leg Deadlifts (Legs #9)
4. Seated or Standing Calves (Legs #11)

Cardiovascular: 20 Minutes, Level 8 exertion

Workout #24

Warm-up:

1. Bike, Treadmill or Elliptical Climber: 5 minutes-Moderate Speed
2. Quadratus Lumborum Stretch (Flexibility #10)
3. Lying Shoulder Clock (Flexibility #4)
4. Triceps Stretch (Flexibility #9)

Resistance Exercises

Perform the same exercise <u>3 consecutive times</u>, 8 to 10 reps. Do not circuit train with power exercises.

1. Barbell High Pull (Upper back #2)
2. Dumbbell Rotator Cuff (Shoulders #6)
3. Dips (Triceps #3) or Bench Dips (Triceps #2)
4. Barbell or EZ "curvy" Bar Standing (Biceps #2)
5. Vertical Knee Raise (Abs #5)

Cardiovascular: 20 Minutes, Level 8 exertion

Week 9—Last week of Power Strength Training.

Workout #25

Warm-up:

1. Bike, Treadmill or Elliptical Climber: 5 minutes-Moderate Speed
2. Hamstring Stretch (Flexibility #1)
3. Lower Back Stretch (Flexibility #2)
4. Shoulder Capsule Stretch (Flexibility #5)

Resistance Exercises

Perform the same exercise <u>3 consecutive times</u>, 8 to 10 reps. Do not circuit train with power exercises.

1. Barbell Power Cleans (Shoulders #1)
2. Barbell Good Mornings (Lower Back #2)
3. Barbell Bench Press (Chest #1)
4. Pullups (Back #4) or Lat-Pulldown Overhand grip (Back #2)
5. Ball Sit up (Abs #4)

Cardiovascular: 20 Minutes, Level 8 exertion

Workout #26

Warm-up:

1. Bike, Treadmill or Elliptical Climber: 5 minutes-Moderate Speed
2. Hamstring Stretch (Flexibility #1)
3. Quadriceps Stretch (Flexibility #3)
4. Gluteus Maximus Stretch (Flexibility #7)

Resistance Exercises

Perform the same exercise 3 consecutive times, 8 to 10 reps. Do not circuit train with power exercises.
1. Barbell Deadlifts (Legs #1)
2. Barbell Squats (Legs #4)
3. Barbell Straight Leg Deadlifts (Legs #9)
4. Seated or Standing Calves (Legs #11)

Cardiovascular: 20 Minutes, Level 8 exertion

Workout #27

Warm-up:

1. Bike, Treadmill or Elliptical Climber: 5 minutes-Moderate Speed
2. Quadratus Lumborum Stretch (Flexibility #10)
3. Lying Shoulder Clock (Flexibility #4)
4. Triceps Stretch (Flexibility #9)

Resistance Exercises

Perform the same exercise 3 consecutive times, 8 to 10 reps. Do not circuit train with power exercises.
1. Barbell High Pull (Upper back #2)
2. Dumbbell Rotator Cuff (Shoulders #6)
3. Dips (Triceps #3) or Bench Dips (Triceps #2)
4. Barbell or EZ "curvy" Bar Standing (Biceps #2)
5. Vertical Knee Raise (Abs #5)

Cardiovascular: 20 Minutes, Level 8 exertion

Congratulations! You are beginning to develop lean muscle tissue. There should be a change in your body fat, muscle tone, strength and energy. Keep up the good work!

Week 10—PHASE II Advanced Level Circuit Training. Goal: Three weeks of muscle shaping and toning employing more repetitions with lighter weight.

Workout #28

Warm-up:

1. Bike, Treadmill or Elliptical Climber: 5 minutes-Moderate Speed
2. Hamstring Stretch (Flexibility #1)
3. Psaos Stretch (Flexibility #6)
4. Standing Chest Stretch (Flexibility #8)

Resistance Exercises

Perform 4 circuits of 12 to 15 repetitions.

1. Barbell Lunges (Legs #5)
2. Hamstring Leg Curls (Legs #8)
3. Dumbbell Swiss Ball Chest Press (Chest #3)
4. Lat Pulldown Overhand (Back #2)
5. Superman (Lower Back #1)
6. Ball Crunch (Abs #1)

Cardiovascular: 25 Minutes, Level 7 exertion

Workout #29

Warm-up:

1. Bike, Treadmill or Elliptical Climber: 5 minutes-Moderate Speed
2. Shoulder Capsule Stretch (Flexibility #5)
3. Tricep Stretch (Flexibility #9)
4. Lying Shoulder Clock Stretch (Flexibility #4)

Resistance Exercises

Perform 4 circuits of 12 to 15 repetitions.

1. Dumbbell Swiss Ball Shoulder Press (Shoulders #5)
2. Dumbbell Lying Tricep Extension "Skull Crushers" (Triceps #1)
3. EZ Bar "curvy" Preacher Curls (Biceps #3)
4. Dumbbell Seated Tricep Extension (Triceps #5)
5. Sit Ups (Abs #2)

Cardiovascular: 25 Minutes, Level 7 exertion

Workout #30

Warm-up:

1. Bike, Treadmill or Elliptical Climber: 5 minutes-Moderate Speed
2. Quadriceps Stretch (Flexibility #3)
3. Lower Back Stretch (Flexibility #2)
4. Standing Chest Stretch (Flexibility #8)

Resistance Exercises

Perform 4 circuits of 12 to 15 repetitions.
1. Barbell Squats (Legs #4)
2. Dumbbell Swiss Ball Chest Press (Chest #3)
3. Dumbbell Step Ups (Legs #7)
4. Dumbbell One Arm Row (Back #3)
5. Barbell Good Morning (Lower Back #2)
6. Twisting Jack Knife (Obliques #2)

Cardiovascular: 25 Minutes, Level 7 exertion

Week 11—PHASE II Advanced Level Circuit Training, continued. Increase the weight while maintaining proper form.

Workout #31

Warm-up:

1. Bike, Treadmill or Elliptical Climber: 5 minutes-Moderate Speed
2. Hamstring Stretch (Flexibility #1)
3. Psaos Stretch (Flexibility #6)
4. Standing Chest Stretch (Flexibility #8)

Resistance Exercises

Perform 4 circuits of 12 to 15 repetitions.
1. Barbell Lunges (Legs #5)
2. Hamstring Leg Curls (Legs #8)
3. Dumbbell Swiss Ball Chest Press (Chest #3)
4. Lat Pulldown Overhand (Back #2)
5. Superman (Lower Back #1)
6. Ball Crunch (Abs #1)

Cardiovascular: 25 Minutes, Level 7 exertion

Workout #32

Warm-up:

1. Bike, Treadmill or Elliptical Climber: 5 minutes-Moderate Speed
2. Shoulder Capsule Stretch (Flexibility #5)
3. Tricep Stretch (Flexibility #9)
4. Lying Shoulder Clock Stretch (Flexibility #4)

Resistance Exercises

Perform 4 circuits of 12 to 15 repetitions.
1. Dumbbell Swiss Ball Shoulder Press (Shoulders #5)
2. Dumbbell Lying Tricep Extension "Skull Crushers" (Triceps #1)
3. EZ Bar "curvy" Preacher Curls (Biceps #3)
4. Dumbbell Seated Tricep Extension (Triceps #5)
5. Sit Ups (Abs #2)

Cardiovascular: 25 Minutes, Level 7 exertion

Workout #33

Warm-up:

1. Bike, Treadmill or Elliptical Climber: 5 minutes-Moderate Speed
2. Quadriceps Stretch (Flexibility #3)
3. Lower Back Stretch (Flexibility #2)
4. Standing Chest Stretch (Flexibility #8)

Resistance Exercises

Perform 4 circuits of 12 to 15 repetitions.
1. Barbell Squats (Legs #4)
2. Dumbbell Swiss Ball Chest Press (Chest #3)
3. Dumbbell Step Ups (Legs #7)
4. Dumbbell One Arm Row (Back #3)
5. Barbell Good Morning (Lower Back #2)
6. Twisting Jack Knife (Obliques #2)

Cardiovascular: 25 Minutes, Level 7 exertion

Week 12—PHASE II Advanced Level Circuit Training, continued. Last week of this phase. Increase the weight while maintaining proper form.

Workout #34

Warm-up:

1. Bike, Treadmill or Elliptical Climber: 5 minutes-Moderate Speed
2. Hamstring Stretch (Flexibility #1)
3. Psaos Stretch (Flexibility #6)
4. Standing Chest Stretch (Flexibility #8)

Resistance Exercises

Perform 4 circuits of 12 to 15 repetitions.

1. Barbell Lunges (Legs #5)
2. Hamstring Leg Curls (Legs #8)
3. Dumbbell Swiss Ball Chest Press (Chest #3)
4. Lat Pulldown Overhand (Back #2)
5. Superman (Lower Back #1)
6. Ball Crunch (Abs #1)

Cardiovascular: 25 Minutes, Level 7 exertion

Workout #35

Warm-up:

1. Bike, Treadmill or Elliptical Climber: 5 minutes-Moderate Speed
2. Shoulder Capsule Stretch (Flexibility #5)
3. Tricep Stretch (Flexibility #9)
4. Lying Shoulder Clock Stretch (Flexibility #4)

Resistance Exercises

Perform 4 circuits of 12 to 15 repetitions.

1. Dumbbell Swiss Ball Shoulder Press (Shoulders #5)
2. Dumbbell Lying Tricep Extension "Skull Crushers" (Triceps #1)
3. EZ "curvy" Bar Preacher Curls (Biceps #3)
4. Bench Dips on Medicine Ball (Triceps #4)
5. Sit Ups (Abs #2)

Cardiovascular: 25 Minutes, Level 7 exertion

Workout #36

Warm-up:

1. Bike, Treadmill or Elliptical Climber: 5 minutes-Moderate Speed
2. Quadriceps Stretch (Flexibility #3)
3. Lower Back Stretch (Flexibility #2)
4. Standing Chest Stretch (Flexibility #8)

Resistance Exercises

Perform 4 circuits of 12 to 15 repetitions.
1. Barbell Squats (Legs #4)
2. Dumbbell Swiss Ball Chest Press (Chest #3)
3. Dumbbell Step Ups (Legs #7)
4. Dumbbell One Arm Row (Back #3)
5. Barbell Good Morning (Lower Back #2)
6. Twisting Jack Knife (Obliques #2)

Cardiovascular: 25 Minutes, Level 7 exertion

Congratulations! You have made it through the fourth segment.

Week 13—Endurance "Interval" Training. Goal: Three weeks of endurance training with shortened rest periods. This will ensure that the metabolism stays fast. The "interval" is reintroduced into the workout, similar to weeks four through six.

Workout #37

Warm-up:

1. Bike, Treadmill or Elliptical Climber: 5 minutes-Moderate Speed
2. Low Back Stretch (Flexibility #2)
3. Psoas Stretch (Flexibility #6)
4. Shoulder Capsule Stretch (Flexibility #5)

Resistance Exercises

Perform 4 circuits of 12 to 15 repetitions.

1. Barbell Bench Press (Chest #1)
2. Dumbbell Incline Chest Press (Chest #5)
3. Interval- Bike/Elliptical/Jump Rope- 45 seconds, fast pace
4. Lat-Pulldown "Neutral Grip" (Back #1)
5. Barbell Bent Over Row (Back #5)
6. Interval- Bike/Elliptical/Jump Rope- 45 seconds, fast pace

Cardiovascular: 30 Minutes, Level 7 exertion

Workout #38

Warm-up:

1. Bike, Treadmill or Elliptical Climber: 5 minutes-Moderate Speed
2. Quadratus Lumborum Stretch (Flexibility #10)
3. Hamstring Stretch (Flexibility #1)
4. Gluteus Maximus Stretch (Flexibility #7)

Resistance Exercises

Perform 4 circuits of 12 to 15 repetitions.

1. Dumbbell Step-ups (Legs #7)
2. Hamstring Leg Curl (Legs #8)
3. Interval- Bike/Elliptical/Jump Rope- 45 seconds, fast pace
4. Swiss Ball Hamstring Bridge (Legs #10)
5. Dumbbell Lunges (Legs #6)
6. Interval- Bike/Elliptical/Jump Rope- 45 seconds, fast pace
7. Twisting Jack Knife (Obliques #2)

Cardiovascular: 30 Minutes, Level 7 exertion

Workout #39

Warm-up:

1. Bike, Treadmill or Elliptical Climber: 5 minutes-Moderate Speed
2. Shoulder Capsule Stretch (Flexibility #5)
3. Tricep Stretch (Flexibility #9)
4. Hamsting Stretch (Flexibility #1)

Resistance Exercises

Perform 4 circuits of 12 to 15 repetitions.

1. Barbell Upright Row (Upper Back #1)
2. Barbell or EZ "curvy" Bar Standing Bicep Curls (Biceps #2)
3. Interval- Bike/Elliptical/Jump Rope- 45 seconds, fast pace
4. Tricep Cable Push Downs (Triceps #6)
5. Dumbbell Rear Lateral Raise (Shoulders #4)
6. Interval- Bike/Elliptical/Jump Rope- 45 seconds, fast pace

Cardiovascular: 30 Minutes, Level 7 exertion

Week 14—Endurance "Interval" Training, continued.

Workout #40

Warm-up:

1. Bike, Treadmill or Elliptical Climber: 5 minutes-Moderate Speed
2. Low Back Stretch (Flexibility #2)
3. Psoas Stretch (Flexibility #6)
4. Shoulder Capsule Stretch (Flexibility #5)

Resistance Exercises

Perform 4 circuits of 12 to 15 repetitions.

1. Barbell Bench Press (Chest #1)
2. Dumbbell Incline Chest Press (Chest #5)
3. Interval- Bike/Elliptical/Jump Rope- 45 seconds, fast pace
4. Lat-Pulldown "Neutral Grip" (Back #1)
5. Barbell Bent Over Row (Back #5)
6. Interval- Bike/Elliptical/Jump Rope- 45 seconds, fast pace

Cardiovascular: 30 Minutes, Level 7 exertion

Workout #41

Warm-up:

1. Bike, Treadmill or Elliptical Climber: 5 minutes-Moderate Speed
2. Quadratus Lumborum Stretch (Flexibility #10)
3. Hamstring Stretch (Flexibility #1)
4. Gluteus Maximus Stretch (Flexibility #7)

Resistance Exercises

Perform 4 circuits of 12 to 15 repetitions.

1. Dumbbell Step-ups (Legs #7)
2. Hamstring Leg Curl (Legs #8)
3. Interval- Bike/Elliptical/Jump Rope- 45 seconds, fast pace
4. Swiss Ball Hamstring Bridge (Legs #10)
5. Dumbbell Lunges (Legs #6)
6. Interval- Bike/Elliptical/Jump Rope- 45 seconds, fast pace
7. Twisting Jack Knife (Obliques #2)

Cardiovascular: 30 Minutes, Level 7 exertion

Workout #42

Warm-up:

1. Bike, Treadmill or Elliptical Climber: 5 minutes-Moderate Speed
2. Shoulder Capsule Stretch (Flexibility #5)
3. Tricep Stretch (Flexibility #9)
4. Hamsting Stretch (Flexibility #1)

Resistance Exercises

Perform 4 circuits of 12 to 15 repetitions.

1. Barbell Upright Row (Upper Back #1)
2. Barbell or EZ "curvy" Bar Standing Bicep Curls (Biceps #2)
3. Interval- Bike/Elliptical/Jump Rope- 45 seconds, fast pace
4. Tricep Cable Push Downs (Triceps #6)
5. Dumbbell Rear Lateral Raise (Shoulders #4)
6. Interval- Bike/Elliptical/Jump Rope- 45 seconds, fast pace

Cardiovascular: 30 Minutes, Level 7 exertion

Week 15—Last week of Endurance "Interval" Training.

Workout #43

Warm-up:

1. Bike, Treadmill or Elliptical Climber: 5 minutes-Moderate Speed
2. Low Back Stretch (Flexibility #2)
3. Psoas Stretch (Flexibility #6)
4. Shoulder Capsule Stretch (Flexibility #5)

Resistance Exercises

Perform 4 circuits of 12 to 15 repetitions.

1. Barbell Bench Press (Chest #1)
2. Dumbbell Incline Chest Press (Chest #5)
3. Interval- Bike/Elliptical/Jump Rope- 45 seconds, fast pace
4. Lat-Pulldown "Neutral Grip" (Back #1)
5. Barbell Bent Over Row (Back #5)
6. Interval- Bike/Elliptical/Jump Rope- 45 seconds, fast pace

Cardiovascular: 30 Minutes, Level 7 exertion

Workout #44

Warm-up:

1. Bike, Treadmill or Elliptical Climber: 5 minutes-Moderate Speed
2. Quadratus Lumborum Stretch (Flexibility #10)
3. Hamstring Stretch (Flexibility #1)
4. Gluteus Maximus Stretch (Flexibility #7)

Resistance Exercises

Perform 4 circuits of 12 to 15 repetitions.

1. Dumbbell Step-ups (Legs #7)
2. Hamstring Leg Curl (Legs #8)
3. Interval- Bike/Elliptical/Jump Rope- 45 seconds, fast pace
4. Swiss Ball Hamstring Bridge (Legs #10)
5. Dumbbell Lunges (Legs #6)
6. Interval- Bike/Elliptical/Jump Rope- 45 seconds, fast pace
7. Twisting Jack Knife (Obliques #2)

Cardiovascular: 30 Minutes, Level 7 exertion

Workout #45

Warm-up:

1. Bike, Treadmill or Elliptical Climber: 5 minutes-Moderate Speed
2. Shoulder Capsule Stretch (Flexibility #5)
3. Tricep Stretch (Flexibility #9)
4. Hamsting Stretch (Flexibility #1)

Resistance Exercises

Perform 4 circuits of 12 to 15 repetitions.
1. Barbell Upright Row (Upper Back #1)
2. Barbell or EZ "curvy" Bar Standing Bicep Curls (Biceps #2)
3. Interval- Bike/Elliptical/Jump Rope- 45 seconds, fast pace
4. Bench Dips on Medicine Ball (Triceps #4)
5. Dumbbell Rear Lateral Raise (Shoulders #4)
6. Interval- Bike/Elliptical/Jump Rope- 45 seconds, fast pace

Cardiovascular: 30 Minutes, Level 7 exertion

Congratulations! You've made it through the fifth segment. Provided your nutrition is supportive, your body is burning fat.

Week 16—Power Strength Training. Goal: Three weeks of strength training focusing on muscle growth. Remember, the more muscle you have, the more body fat you will burn.

Workout #46

Warm-up:

1. Bike, Treadmill or Elliptical Climber: 5 minutes-Moderate Speed
2. Hamstring Stretch (Flexibility #1)
3. Low Back Stretch (Flexibility #2)
4. Shoulder Capsule Stretch (Flexibility #5)

Resistance Exercises

Perform the same exercise <u>4 consecutive times</u>, 8 to 10 reps. Do not circuit train with power exercises.
1. Barbell Power Cleans (Shoulders #1)
2. Barbell Good Mornings (Lower Back #2)
3. Barbell Bench Press (Chest #1)
4. Pullups (Back #4) or Lat-Pulldown "Overhand Grip" (Back #2)
5. Ball Sit Up (Abs #4)

Cardiovascular: 20 Minutes, Level 8 exertion

Workout #47

Warm-up:

1. Bike, Treadmill or Elliptical Climber: 5 minutes-Moderate Speed
2. Hamstring Stretch (Flexibility #1)
3. Quadriceps Stretch (Flexibility #3)
4. Gluteus Maximus Stretch (Flexibility #7)

Resistance Exercises

Perform the same exercise 4 consecutive times, 8 to 10 reps. Do not circuit train with power exercises.

1. Barbell Deadlifts (Legs #1)
2. Barbell Squats (Legs #4)
3. Barbell Straight Leg Deadlifts (Legs #9)
4. Seated or Standing Calves (Legs #11)

Cardiovascular: 20 Minutes, Level 8 exertion

Workout #48

Warm-up:

1. Bike, Treadmill or Elliptical Climber: 5 minutes-Moderate Speed
2. Quadratus Lumborum Stretch (Flexibility #10)
3. Lying Shoulder Clock (Flexibility #4)
4. Triceps Stretch (Flexibility #9)

Resistance Exercises

Perform the same exercise 4 consecutive times, 8 to 10 reps. Do not circuit train with power exercises.

1. Barbell High Pull (Upper back #2)
2. Barbell Push Press (Shoulders #2)
3. Dips (Triceps #3) or Bench Dips (Triceps #2)
4. Barbell or EZ "curvy" Bar Standing (Biceps #2)
5. Vertical Knee Raise (Abs #5)

Cardiovascular: 20 Minutes, Level 8 exertion

Week 17—Power Strength Training, continued. Remember, the more muscle you have, the more body fat you will burn.

Workout #49

Warm-up:

1. Bike, Treadmill or Elliptical Climber: 5 minutes-Moderate Speed
2. Hamstring Stretch (Flexibility #1)
3. Low Back Stretch (Flexibility #2)
4. Shoulder Capsule Stretch (Flexibility #5)

Resistance Exercises

Perform the same exercise 4 consecutive times, 8 to 10 reps. Do not circuit train with power exercises.
1. Barbell Power Cleans (Shoulders #1)
2. Barbell Good Mornings (Lower Back #2)
3. Barbell Bench Press (Chest #1)
4. Pullups (Back #4) or Lat-Pulldown "Overhand Grip" (Back #2)
5. Ball Sit Up (Abs #4)

Cardiovascular: 20 Minutes, Level 8 exertion

Workout #50

Warm-up:

1. Bike, Treadmill or Elliptical Climber: 5 minutes-Moderate Speed
2. Hamstring Stretch (Flexibility #1)
3. Quadriceps Stretch (Flexibility #3)
4. Gluteus Maximus Stretch (Flexibility #7)

Resistance Exercises

Perform the same exercise 4 consecutive times, 8 to 10 reps. Do not circuit train with power exercises.
1. Barbell Deadlifts (Legs #1)
2. Barbell Squats (Legs #4)
3. Barbell Straight Leg Deadlifts (Legs #9)
4. Seated or Standing Calves (Legs #11)

Cardiovascular: 20 Minutes, Level 8 exertion

Workout #51

Warm-up:

1. Bike, Treadmill or Elliptical Climber: 5 minutes-Moderate Speed
2. Quadratus Lumborum Stretch (Flexibility #10)
3. Lying Shoulder Clock (Flexibility #4)
4. Triceps Stretch (Flexibility #9)

Resistance Exercises

Perform the same exercise 4 consecutive times, 8 to 10 reps. Do not circuit train with power exercises.

1. Barbell High Pull (Upper back #2)
2. Barbell Push Press (Shoulders #2)
3. Dips (Triceps #3) or Bench Dips (Triceps #2)
4. Barbell or EZ "curvy" Bar Standing (Biceps #2)
5. Vertical Knee Raise (Abs #5)

Cardiovascular: 20 Minutes, Level 8 exertion

Week 18—Last week of Power Strength Training.

Workout #52

Warm-up:

1. Bike, Treadmill or Elliptical Climber: 5 minutes-Moderate Speed
2. Hamstring Stretch (Flexibility #1)
3. Low Back Stretch (Flexibility #2)
4. Shoulder Capsule Stretch (Flexibility #5)

Resistance Exercises

Perform the same exercise 4 consecutive times, 8 to 10 reps. Do not circuit train with power exercises.

1. Barbell Power Cleans (Shoulders #1)
2. Barbell Good Mornings (Lower Back #2)
3. Barbell Bench Press (Chest #1)
4. Pullups (Back #4) or Lat-Pulldown "Overhand Grip" (Back #2)
5. Ball Sit Up (Abs #4)

Cardiovascular: 20 Minutes, Level 8 exertion

Workout #53

Warm-up:

1. Bike, Treadmill or Elliptical Climber: 5 minutes-Moderate Speed
2. Hamstring Stretch (Flexibility #1)
3. Quadriceps Stretch (Flexibility #3)
4. Gluteus Maximus Stretch (Flexibility #7)

Resistance Exercises

Perform the same exercise 4 consecutive times, 8 to 10 reps. Do not circuit train with power exercises.

1. Barbell Deadlifts (Legs #1)
2. Barbell Squats (Legs #4)
3. Barbell Straight Leg Deadlifts (Legs #9)
4. Seated or Standing Calves (Legs #11)

Cardiovascular: 20 Minutes, Level 8 exertion

Workout #54

Warm-up:

1. Bike, Treadmill or Elliptical Climber: 5 minutes-Moderate Speed
2. Quadratus Lumborum Stretch (Flexibility #10)
3. Lying Shoulder Clock (Flexibility #4)
4. Triceps Stretch (Flexibility #9)

Resistance Exercises

Perform the same exercise 4 consecutive times, 8 to 10 reps. Do not circuit train with power exercises.

1. Barbell High Pull (Upper back #2)
2. Barbell Push Press (Shoulders #2)
3. Dips (Triceps #3) or Bench Dips (Triceps #2)
4. Barbell or EZ "curvy" Bar Standing (Biceps #2)
5. Vertical Knee Raise (Abs #5)

Cardiovascular: 20 Minutes, Level 8 exertion

Congratulations! You have made it through the sixth segment. There should be a change in your body fat, muscle tone, strength and energy. You can now either go back to workout #1 and perform the same workouts with increased weights or go to www.Alessifit.com and order a different workout.

Never Stop Exercising and Lose Fat Forever!

Chart Your Progress

Warm Up

1. Bike
2. Treadmill
3. Elliptical

Flexibility

1. Hamstrings
2. Lower Back
3. Quadriceps
4. Lying Shoulder Clock
5. Shoulder Capsule
6. Psoas
7. Gluteus Maximus
8. Standing Chest Stretch
9. Triceps
10. Quadratus Lumborum

Abs

1. Ball Crunch
2. Sit Up
3. Hip Extension-Supine
4. Swiss Ball Crunches
5. Vertical Knee Raise

Obliques

1. Swiss Ball Twists
2. Twisting Jack Knife

Back

1. Lat Pull-Down "Neutral Grip"
2. Lat Pull –Down "Overhand Grip"
3. Dumbbell One Arm Rows
4. Pull-up
5. Barbell Bent Over Rows
6. Seated Cable Rows

Upper Back

1. Upright Rows
2. High Pull

Lower Back

1. Superman
2. Barbell Good Mornings

Legs

1. Barbell Deadlifts
2. Dumbbell Split Squats
3. Swiss Ball Squats
4. Barbell Squats
5. Barbell Lunges
6. Dumbbell Lunges
7. Dumbbell Step-ups
8. Hamstring Leg Curl
9. Barbell Straight Leg Deadlift
10. Swiss Ball Hamstring Bridge
11. Seated or Standing Calf Raises

Chest

1. Barbell Bench Press
2. Dumbbell Chest Press
3. Dumbbell Swiss Ball Bench Press
4. Dumbbell Chest Fly
5. Dumbbell Incline Chest Press

Shoulders

1. Barbell Power Cleans
2. Barbell Push Press
3. Dumbbell Shoulder Press
4. Dumbbell Rear Lateral Raise
5. Dumbbell Swiss Ball Shoulder Press
6. Dumbbell Rotator Cuff

Biceps

1. Dumbbell Standing Hammer Curls
2. Barbell or EZ bar Standing Curl

3. EZ bar Preacher Curl
4. Dumbbell Seated Alternating Bicep Curls

Triceps

1. Dumbbell Lying Tricep Extension "Skull Crushers"
2. Bench Dips
3. Dips
4. Bench Dips, feet on medicine ball
5. Dumbbell Seated Tricep Extension
6. Tricep Cable Pushdowns

22

MAINTAIN YOUR SUCCESS

Congratulations! How does it feel? You've proven your commitment to your health and fitness and are now enjoying the benefits. Does it feel better or worse to have more muscle tone?

Do you like carrying more body fat or less? How does it feel to have energy and stamina throughout the day? Do you enjoy fitting into clothes that were too tight only eighteen weeks ago? Do you have any desire to go back to your previous unhealthy lifestyle with less muscle tone, more body fat and fewer health benefits?

I believe every person has it within his- or herself to dramatically transform their lives and improve their health and fitness. I never question a person's ability; I only question their commitment. If you've made it to this page in the book, you've demonstrated your commitment.

You may be asking yourself, "What do I do now that I have completed the eighteen weeks?" The answer is to continue your healthy lifestyle and *repeat* the Lose Fat Forever system. You know how this system works—I want you to do it again. I want you to repeat the workouts from week one to week eighteen. However, the second time through, I want you to increase the intensity of your workouts by increasing the weights. As I mentioned previously, your body needs new stimuli in order to develop and maintain lean muscle tone. Now that you've developed strength and lean muscle tone, you need to increase the challenge to your body. Increasing weights during the workout will meet this need.

Only use weights within your capabilities. Don't risk injury by using weights that are *too* heavy. If you have any questions on how much weight to use for various exercises, please contact a personal fitness professional.

I have used this eighteen-week program with my clients for years while maintaining and developing lean muscle tissue. The program doesn't stagnate because it changes virtually every workout. I'm able to continue to stimulate clients' lean muscle tissue because I increase weights as they develop strength.

You can use the eighteen-week workout indefinitely provided you keep challenging your lean muscle tissue with increased weights. If you feel a need to do a completely different workout routine, you can visit our website, www.AlessiFit.com.

Now that you have lowered your body fat, you may either want to lower it further or maintain your current level. In order to do this, you will need to continue to weight train, eat supportive meals and perform moderate cardiovascular training. By now, you know that a supportive meal is a lean protein, a slow-releasing carbohydrate and a green vegetable. Your meal frequency should still be every three to three and a half hours with serving sizes as large as your clenched fist. You'll need to continue to eat in this manner six days a week. The seventh day should still be your cheat day; enjoy yourself and eat whatever you want, in moderation.

Now that you have begun to feel the positive benefits of a healthier, fit lifestyle, I know you'll want to keep it up. You've come so far and you should be proud of yourself. As I say to my clients, "If you aren't careful, you might actually feel better and live longer!" I hope you also feel better and live longer. Good luck!

GLOSSARY

Adipose: Body fat.

Aerobic: Means "with oxygen." Occurs during low intensity exercise like walking. In this system, it is important to perform in moderation.

Alcohol: Any intoxicating liquor.

Amino acid: A group of compounds that are the building blocks of protein and muscle.

Anaerobic: Means "without oxygen." Occurs in high-intensity activities like sprinting or weight lifting. Anaerobic exercise and developing muscle tissue is the best and quickest way to increase metabolism and reduce body fat.

Atrophy: A wasting away, or decrease in the size of muscle tissue, usually from lack of use. Atrophy can occur as quickly as forty-eight hours post-workout.

Blood sugar (glucose): Sugar in the blood, usually formed from carbohydrates.

Body fat: The accumulation of adipose tissue. Body fat is usually measured in a percentage and varies according to age and gender. One of the goals of this system is to help reduce body fat.

Burning (calories): The rate at which your body utilizes fuel, either muscle, fat or glycogen.

Calories: The amount of heat required to raise one kilogram of water one degree Celsius.

Cannibalization: The detrimental effect of breaking down lean muscle tissue to get energy or essential fatty acids.

Carbohydrate: A macronutrient composed of carbon, hydrogen and oxygen. An effective fuel source for the body. Includes starches, sugars and fibers. One gram of carbohydrates equals four calories.

Cardiovascular diseases: Diseases of the heart and blood vessels.

Cardiovascular training: A type of aerobic training that is of low intensity and long duration.

Cheat day: The one day per week you can eat whatever you like, in moderation.

Circuit training: A method of resistance training that employs the use of multiple exercises performed one after another. Usually utilizes moderately lighter weight with more repetitions.

Complex carbohydrate (polysaccharides): Composed of many monosaccharides (simple sugars). Complex carbohydrates provide energy for the body and brain. They have a higher thermal effect than simple carbohydrates.

Craving: Extreme desire, mostly from sugar or fat products.

Diabetes: A metabolism disease in which carbohydrate use is reduced and lipid and protein use is enhanced; caused by deficiency or lack of insulin. The body no longer effectively regulates blood sugar.

Diet: Short-term nutritional pattern in which calories are reduced. Not an effective way to lose fat.

Diet drugs: Both over-the-counter and prescription drugs designed to make you feel satiated (full). Over time, these drugs condition the metabolism to work slower when muscle tissue is decreased.

Endurance training: Done to sustain energy over a period of time. It is usually anaerobic such as weight lifting or sprinting.

Essential fatty acids: Fats the body cannot make, which must be obtained from food. These fats are important to cellular synthesis and hormone production. Flaxseed oil, fish oil and safflower oil are good sources of these fats.

Fast-releasing carbohydrate: Carbohydrates or sugars that increase blood sugar quickly. This rise is usually followed by a surge in insulin secretion. Examples include mono- and disaccharides such as fruit (fructose) and table sugar (sucrose).

Fat: One of the macronutrients, some of which are essential to carry out body processes. There are two types of fats, saturated (bad) and unsaturated (good).

Fat blockers: Prescription and over-the-counter medicine claiming to block saturated dietary fat from being stored in the body as body fat. These products will not work.

Fat oxidation: Reduction or burning of body fat.

Food manufacturers: Companies that make food products to sell in the marketplace.

Glucagon: A hormone secreted from the islets of Langerhans in the pancreas; acts primarily on the liver to release glucose into the blood. Also aids in the burning of fat.

Glycogen: A sugar formed from glucose that is stored in the muscle. These stores are used for energy and, when the stores are full, the muscles look and feel hard.

Hydration: Proper intake of water for cells of the body to be healthy.

Hydrogenated: A fat that is solid at room temperature. These fats include margarine and peanut butter, and should be limited.

Hypertension: High blood pressure.

Insulin: A hormone secreted by the pancreas that increases the uptake of glucose and amino acids by most tissues.

Labeling laws: Laws that stipulate the information that food manufacturers must include on the labels of their products. These laws have loopholes that food manufacturers can manipulate, for example, serving size.

Lipid: Usually refers to fats.

Low calorie diet: Short-term nutritional plan that is designed to limit calories so that scale weight (mostly water) can be reduced. These diets often have a negative impact on metabolism.

Macronutrient: Groups of foods that include proteins, carbohydrates and fats. Chemicals taken into the body that are used to produce energy, provide building blocks for new molecules or function in other chemical reactions.

Meal replacement shakes: Engineered foods that contain carbohydrates, protein and fats in liquid form.

Metabolism: The rate or speed at which the body processes food.

Misinformation: Information that is deceptive and misleading.

Mitochondria: Small rod shape or spherical structures in the muscles that are the site of heat and energy production and in which fat and calories are burned.

Moderate cardiovascular training: Performing a limited amount of aerobic training so that muscle is not broken down by the body for energy.

Muscle tissue: One of the four major tissue types, characterized by its contractile abilities.

Nourishment: Substances that are ingested and digested to maintain life and growth.

Obese: Excessively fat.

Periodization: A term personal trainers use for workout variation.

Plateau: A period of little positive change in the body while exercising. Usually has to do with lack of body fat reduction.

Post-workout: The period of time, usually up to forty minutes after the workout, when glycogen stores are depleted and muscle tissue is broken down.

Protein: Macronutrient consisting of long sequences of amino acids linked together by peptide bonds. Protein is the building block of muscle and has the highest thermal effect of any macronutrient.

Protein bars: Manufactured candy bars that claim to contain high amounts of protein and few carbohydrates and sugars.

Protein day: A nutritional approach designed to hasten the reduction of body fat. Should be done only on non-weight training days. Lean protein sources and vegetable should still be consumed.

Protein drinks: Synthetically manufactured protein, usually from whey or egg sources, designed to help repair muscle tissue after a workout.

Quick fix syndrome: Many Americans continuously jeopardize their health and fitness because they are unwilling to spend the necessary time to perform a complete program. They want quick results and often buy products that can be harmful or engage in a low calorie diet that slows their metabolism further.

Satiation: Feeling satisfied. Essential fatty acids satisfy the body's desire to consume foods rich in fat or sugar.

Saturated fats: Fatty acid in which the carbon chain contains only single bonds between carbon atoms. These are "bad" fats. Examples include cheese, butter, pork and palm oil.

Scale weight: The sum of your muscle, bone, water and fat expressed in pounds or kilograms. This number tells nothing of a person's body composition.

Serving size: The suggested amount or portion that food manufacturers indicate on the labels of their products. Many times this amount is extremely small.

Simple carbohydrate: A mono- or disaccharide. Includes glucose, fruit (fructose) and table sugar (sucrose). Tends to elevate blood sugar quickly.

Slow-releasing carbohydrate: Complex carbohydrates that don't quickly spike blood sugar levels because of the time it takes the body to chemically break down these sugars into glucose. Wheat bread, sweet potatoes and brown rice are examples.

Starch: Carbohydrates. Found in plants, are long chains of glucose molecules. Examples include bread, rice and potatoes.

Starving: Occurs when the body doesn't receive adequate fuel, as on various diets. It economizes and burns less fuel, thus the metabolism is conditioned to burn more slowly.

Strength training: Type of weight training that generally combines more weight with fewer repetitions.

Supplementation: Means "in addition to" not "instead of." Supplements can be used to enhance the results attained through proper nutrition and regular workouts.

Supportive foods: As used in this system, describes various types of foods that will help to build muscle, sustain energy and burn fat. They include lean protein sources, slow-releasing carbohydrates and vegetables.

Sweet tooth: The physical and psychological cravings that occur in response to sugary or high carbohydrate foods that cause a spike in blood sugar. The body releases insulin to stabilize the blood sugar level, which often dips below the normal range. The body then craves more sugar to elevate the levels to normal.

Synergy: A term used in this system to demonstrate how the combined effect of developing lean muscle tissue, eating supportive meals frequently and performing a moderate amount of cardiovascular training is greater compared to any component alone.

Thermal effect of food: The calories or energy required to process and burn food. Protein has the highest effect, carbohydrates are in the middle and fat has the lowest thermal effect.

Transform: A way to dramatically change a person's health and fitness.

Type two diabetes (mellitus): Also referred to as adult onset. Metabolic disease in which carbohydrate use is reduced and that of lipid and protein is enhanced; caused by deficiency of insulin.

Unsaturated fats: Monounsaturated includes olive and peanut oils while polyunsaturated includes flax, safflower and fish oils. These are "good" fats.

Variation: Refers to constantly changing workouts (periodization) for ongoing progress.

Weight-training (resistance): The use of free weights, body weight or machines to create force on muscle tissue. This is the most effective way to develop lean muscle tissue, increase metabolism and reduce body fat.

SOURCES OF INFORMATION

1. American Diabetes Association. 1999 Annual Report.

2. American Heart Association. "Fiber, Lipid, and Coronary Heart Disease." *A Statement for Health Care Professionals From the Nutrition Committee*, American Heart Association, 1997.

3. Boyles, S. *WebMD Medical News*. "Looking for the Fountain of Youth? Try the Gym." September 2001.

4. Bouchard, Claude. *Physical Activity and Obesity*. Baton Rouge: Human Kinetics Publishing Inc., 2000.

5. Centers for Disease Control and Prevention. "Obesity and Overweight: A Public Health Epidemic." Online media. September, 2001.

6. Centers for Disease Control and Prevention. "Prevalence of Healthy Lifestyle Characteristics-Michigan, 1998-2000." Online media. September 2001.

7. Cigolini, M., G. Targher, A.I.A. Bergamo, M. Tonoli, F. Filippi, M. Muggeo, and G. De Sandre. "Moderate alcohol consumption and its relation to visceral fat and plasma androgens in healthy women." *International Journal of Obesity* 20:206–212, 1996.

8. Colino, S. *Self.com*. "Eat Well: The Health Payoffs of Mini Meals." March 2001.

9. Foreyt, J.P. and K. Goodrick. "The ultimate triumph of obesity." *The Lancet* 346: 134–135, 1995.

10. Forte, J. "Vegetarians Versus Meat Eaters." *Personal Fitness Professional*, September 2001.

11. *Health.com*. "Squeeze in Fitness." September 2001.

12. Kaplan, P. *The Answer*. "Personal Development." 1999.

13. Karas, J. *Business Plan for the Body*. New York: Three Rivers Press, 2001.

14. Kuzemchak, S. *Shape Magazine*. "Small Changes, Big Payoffs." April 2001.

15. Mayo Clinic. "Obesity." May 2001.

16. *Men's Fitness*. "23 Essential Tips for Gaining Muscle." May 2001.

17. O'Shea, M. *Parade Magazine*. "Better Fitness." September 16, 2001.

18. Philips, B. *Body for Life*. New York: Harper Collins, 1999.

19. Pollan, Michael. "When a Crop Becomes King," New York Times Online, July 20, 2002.

20. Porcari, John P., McLean. Karen Palmer. et al. "Effects of Electrical Muscle Stimulation on Body Composition, Muscle Strength, and Physical Appearance," *Journal of Strength and Conditioning Research*, 2002, 16(2), 165-172.

21. Ryttig K.R., G. Tellnes, L. Haegh, E. Boe, H. Fagerthun. "A dietary fiber supplement and weight maintenance after weight reduction: a randomized, double blind, placebo controlled long-term trial." *International Journal of Obesity* 13:165–171, 1989.

22. Stunkard, A., Wadden T. *Obesity: Theory and Therapy*. New York: Raven Press, 1993.

23. Tremblay, A., E. Wouters, M. Wenker, S. St-Pierre, C. Bouchard, and J.P. Despres. "Alcohol and high fat diet: a combination favoring overfeeding." *American Journal of Clinical Nutrition* 62:639–644, 1995.

24. Trubo, Richard. "Nutrition Bars: Healthy or Hype?" WebMD, July 15, 2002.

25. Vitetta-Miller, R. *Shape Magazine*. "Eggs For Dinner." March 2001.

26. Vitetta-Miller, R. *Shape Magazine*. "Rise and Dine." May 2001.

27. Walters, Peter Hudson, Ph.D. "Sleep, the Athlete, and Performance," *Strength & Conditioning Journal*, Volume 24, Number 2:17-24, April 2002.

28. Whitaker, R.C., J.A. Wright, M.S. Pepe, K.D. Seidel, and W.H. Dietz. "Predicting obesity in young adulthood from childhood and parental obesity." *New England Journal of Medicine* 337:869–873, 1997.

29. www.ArtToday.com. Stock art.

Recommended Supplements

I am asked all the time what types and brands of supplements I recommend. While there are a small number of quality supplement manufacturers, most are inferior. I often recommend a few key supplements from a company named Human Development Technologies (HDT). I have included their information below. In my experience, I have found HDT to offer superior products at reasonable prices. Here are the supplements I recommend.

Pro Blend 55 (Protein Powder)

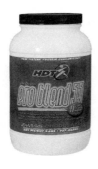

The primary supplement that is essential to gaining lean muscle tissue and decreasing body fat is protein powder. Remember, your body needs protein to repair muscle tissue and increase your metabolism. The more types of protein you consume, the better the protein will absorb into your body. Pro Blend contains a unique blend of proteins, (including micro ultra filtered whey, ion exchanged whey, hydrolyzed whey, egg albumen, and micellar cassein). Pro-Blend's great taste is low in fat, lactose free, aspartame free and mixes instantly in water with no clumping. It comes in 4 flavors; chocolate, vanilla, strawberry and mocha cappuccino.

Fiber Psyll (Fiber)

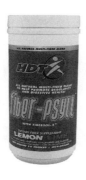

Americans don't eat enough green vegetables and primarily get their fiber from poor sources like enriched white flour and grains. The American Heart Association recommends consuming a combination of 25 to 30 grams of soluble and insoluble fiber a day. In addition to eating green vegetables and slow releasing carbohydrates, it is important to supplement with fiber. However, most fiber supplements have a gritty and unpleasant taste. FIBER-Psyll has a pleasant citrus flavor with a subtle pulp texture. FIBER-Psyll also helps reduce blood serum cholesterol, blood triglycerides, and aids in digestion.

L-Glutamine

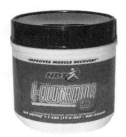

L-Glutamine is an amino acid and is important in its ability to repair and recuperate muscle tissue. L-Glutamine is also vital in allowing your immune system to operate effectively and helps prevent illnesses. L-Glutamine levels are depleted under times of stress such as intense exercise, emotional stress or trauma from surgery. Intense weight training has been shown to suppress the immune system. When stressed, the cells of the immune system require more L-Glutamine than the body can manufacture. I recommend you add L-Glutamine to your post-workout protein drink (ProBlend 55) each workout. This will ensure you are helping to repair your muscle tissue and protect your immune system.

Solid Gains

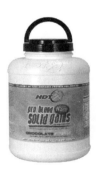

For those of you who are looking to gain muscle and are not concerned with losing body fat, use Solid Gains. Solid Gains contains a blended protein matrix similar to Pro Blend 55, along with optimum ratios of carbohydrates and fats, 11 grams of branch chain amino acids and 3 grams of essential fatty acids from flax seeds. Solid Gains includes a time-released blend of whey protein isolates, egg protein and milk protein to deliver 60 grams of protein per serving which is aspartame free. Solid Gains also delivers 100 grams of carbohydrates with only 6 grams of sugar. A great post workout supplement as well.

MD Labs & Human Development Technologies
3925 E. Watkins
Suite 200
Phoenix, AZ 85034
Phone: (800) 927-1034
www.mdlabs.com

Order Form

📠 **Fax orders:** (716) 633-2030. Fax this form.

💻 **E-mail orders:** ThePromise@alessifit.com

Website: www.AlessiFit.com

✉ **Mail orders:**   **Alessi Fitness**
                                   7662 Transit Road
                                   Williamsville, NY 14221 USA

Please send me the following:

❏ *Lose Fat Forever* book $15.95

❏ *The Promise Fat Loss & Fitness System* hardcover book $25.95

❏ *The Promise Fat Loss & Fitness System* audio 2 disk CD $15.95

Name: _____

Address: _____

City, State, Zip: _____

Telephone: _____

E-mail address: _____

Sales tax: Please add 8% for New York residents

Shipping by air:
    US: $5 for the first book or disk and $2 for each additional product.
    International: $10 for first book or disk and $6 for each additional product

Payment: ❏ Visa   ❏ MasterCard   ❏ American Express
                ❏ Discover

Card number: _____

Name on card: _____ Exp. Date: _____

Card holder signature: _____

- **Interactive e-mail service**

Go to www.AlessiFit.com to find out how you can become a client of the Alessi brothers no matter where you live! Interact with Derek & Don Alessi for all of your fitness and nutrition needs. The interactive e-mail service allows you to ask questions directly to the fitness experts with regards to your personal goals.

- **Interactive e-mail service for personal trainers**

Personal Trainers can now utilize the Alessi brothers' knowledge and experience to help your own business flourish. The Alessi's have been mentoring elite-level trainers for years and now you too can share their wisdom and learn how to get astonishing results with your clients. This is an essential tool in becoming the most in-demand trainer in your area. Go to www.AlessiFit.com for details.

Order Form

📠 **Fax orders:** (716) 633-2030. Fax this form.

💻 **E-mail orders:** ThePromise@alessifit.com

Website: www.AlessiFit.com

✉ **Mail orders:**   **Alessi Fitness**
7662 Transit Road
Williamsville, NY 14221 USA

Please send me the following:

❏ *Lose Fat Forever* book $15.95

❏ *The Promise Fat Loss & Fitness System* hardcover book $25.95

❏ *The Promise Fat Loss & Fitness System* audio 2 disk CD $15.95

Name: _____

Address: _____

City, State, Zip: _____

Telephone: _____

E-mail address: _____

Sales tax: Please add 8% for New York residents

Shipping by air:
US: $5 for the first book or disk and $2 for each additional product.
International: $10 for first book or disk and $6 for each additional product

Payment: ❏ Visa   ❏ MasterCard   ❏ American Express
❏ Discover

Card number: _____

Name on card: _____ Exp. Date: _____

Card holder signature: _____

- **Interactive e-mail service**

Go to www.AlessiFit.com to find out how you can become a client of the Alessi brothers no matter where you live! Interact with Derek & Don Alessi for all of your fitness and nutrition needs. The interactive e-mail service allows you to ask questions directly to the fitness experts with regards to your personal goals.

- **Interactive e-mail service for personal trainers**

Personal Trainers can now utilize the Alessi brothers' knowledge and experience to help your own business flourish. The Alessi's have been mentoring elite-level trainers for years and now you too can share their wisdom and learn how to get astonishing results with your clients. This is an essential tool in becoming the most in-demand trainer in your area. Go to www.AlessiFit.com for details.